Care of the Cirrhotic Patient

Guest Editor

DAVID A. SASS, MD

MEDICAL CLINICS OF NORTH AMERICA

www.medical.theclinics.com

July 2009 • Volume 93 • Number 4

SAUNDERS an imprint of ELSEVIER, Inc.

W.B. SAUNDERS COMPANY
A Division of Elsevier Inc.

1600 John F. Kennedy Boulevard • Suite 1800 • Philadelphia, Pennsylvania 19103-2899

http://www.theclinics.com

MEDICAL CLINICS OF NORTH AMERICA Volume 93, Number 4
July 2009 ISSN 0025-7125, ISBN-13: 978-1-4377-1240-7, ISBN-10: 1-4377-1240-1

Editor: Rachel Glover
Developmental Editor: Donald Mumford

Medical Clinics of North America (ISSN 0025-7125) is published bimonthly by W.B. Saunders, 360 Park Avenue South, New York, NY 10010-1710. Business and editorial offices: 1600 John F. Kennedy Boulevard, Suite 1800, Philadelphia, PA 19103-2899. Accounting and circulation offices: 6277 Sea Harbor Drive, Orlando, FL 32887-4800. Periodicals postage paid at New York, NY, and additional mailing offices. Subscription prices are USD 187 per year for US individuals, USD 334 per year for US institutions, USD 96 per year for US students, USD 238 per year for Canadian individuals, USD 434 per year for Canadian institutions, USD 151 per year for Canadian students, USD 288 per year for international individuals, USD 434 per year for international institutions and USD 151 per year for international students. To receive student/resident rate, orders must be accompanied by name of affiliated institution, date of term, and the *signature* of program/residency coordinator on institution letterhead. Orders will be billed at individual rate until proof of status is received. Foreign air speed delivery is included in all *Clinics* subscription prices. All prices are subject to change without notice. POSTMASTER: Send address changes to *Medical Clinics of North America*, Elsevier Periodicals Customer Service, 11830 Westline Industrial Drive, St. Louis, MO 63146. Customer Service (orders, claims, online, change of address): Elsevier Periodicals Customer Service, 11830 Westline Industrial Drive, St. Louis, MO 63146. Tel: 1-800-654-2452 (U.S. and Canada); 314-453-7041 (outside U.S. and Canada). Fax: 314-453-5170. E-mail: journalscustomerservice-usa@elsevier.com (for print support); journalsonlinesupport-usa@elsevier.com (for online support).

Reprints. For copies of 100 or more of articles in this publication, please contact the Commercial Reprints Department, Elsevier Inc., 360 Park Avenue South, New York, NY 10010-1710. Tel.: 212-633-3812; Fax: 212-462-1935; E-mail: reprints@elsevier.com.

Medical Clinics of North America is also published in Spanish by McGraw-Hill Interamericana Editores S. A., P.O. Box 5-237, 06500 Mexico, D.F., Mexico.

Medical Clinics of North America is covered in *MEDLINE/PubMed (Index Medicus), Current Contents, ASCA, Excerpta Medica, Science Citation Index,* and *ISI/BIOMED.*

Printed in the United States of America.

GOAL STATEMENT

The goal of *Medical Clinics of North America* is to keep practicing physicians up to date with current clinical practice by providing timely articles reviewing the state of the art in patient care.

ACCREDITATION

The *Medical Clinics of North America* is planned and implemented in accordance with the Essential Areas and Policies of the Accreditation Council for Continuing Medical Education (ACCME) through the joint sponsorship of the University of Virginia School of Medicine and Elsevier. The University of Virginia School of Medicine is accredited by the ACCME to provide continuing medical education for physicians.

The University of Virginia School of Medicine designates this educational activity for a maximum of 15 *AMA PRA Category 1 Credits*™ for each issue, 90 credits per year. Physicians should only claim credit commensurate with the extent of their participation in the activity.

The American Medical Association has determined that physicians not licensed in the US who participate in this CME activity are eligible for a maximum of 15 *AMA PRA Category 1 Credits*™ for each issue, 90 credits per year.

Credit can be earned by reading the text material, taking the CME examination online at http://www.theclinics.com/home/cme, and completing the evaluation. After taking the test, you will be required to review any and all incorrect answers. Following completion of the test and evaluation, your credit will be awarded and you may print your certificate.

FACULTY DISCLOSURE/CONFLICT OF INTEREST

The University of Virginia School of Medicine, as an ACCME accredited provider, endorses and strives to comply with the Accreditation Council for Continuing Medical Education (ACCME) Standards of Commercial Support, Commonwealth of Virginia statutes, University of Virginia policies and procedures, and associated federal and private regulations and guidelines on the need for disclosure and monitoring of proprietary and financial interests that may affect the scientific integrity and balance of content delivered in continuing medical education activities under our auspices.

The University of Virginia School of Medicine requires that all CME activities accredited through this institution be developed independently and be scientifically rigorous, balanced and objective in the presentation/discussion of its content, theories and practices.

All authors/editors participating in an accredited CME activity are expected to disclose to the readers relevant financial relationships with commercial entities occurring within the past 12 months (such as grants or research support, employee, consultant, stock holder, member of speakers bureau, etc.). The University of Virginia School of Medicine will employ appropriate mechanisms to resolve potential conflicts of interest to maintain the standards of fair and balanced education to the reader. Questions about specific strategies can be directed to the Office of Continuing Medical Education, University of Virginia School of Medicine, Charlottesville, Virginia.

The faculty and staff of the University of Virginia Office of Continuing Medical Education have no financial affiliations to disclose.

The authors/editors listed below have identified no professional or financial affiliations for themselves or their spouse/partner:

Jawad Ahmad, MD, MRCP; Zygimantas C. Alsauskas, MD; Kapil B. Chopra, MD, DM, FACP; Matthew S. Cohen, MD; Juan F. Gallegos-Orozco, MD; Rachel Glover (Acquisitions Editor); Wei Hou, MD; Harvey B. Lefton, MD; Lina Mackelaite, MD; Shahid M. Malik, MD; Gaurav Mehta, MD; Manuel Mendizabal, MD; Anthony Rosa, MD; Charandpal Singh, MD; Vinay Sundaram, MD; Hugo E. Vargas, MD; and Andrew Wolf, MD (Test Author).

The authors/editors listed below identified the following professional or financial affiliations for themselves or their spouse/partner:

Karthik Ranganna, MD is an industry funded research/investigator for Wyeth Pharmaceuticals.

K. Rajender Reddy, MD is an industry funded research/investigator for Roche, Vertex, and Gilead, serves on the Speakers Bureau for Roche, serves on the Advisory Committee for Roche, Vertex, Gilead, and Salix, and has received other support from NIH/NIDDK, NIH/NIDDK, NIH/FDA, NIH/NCCAM, University of Michigan, Virginia Commonwealth University, NIH/FDA, University of California- San Francisco, and University of Texas.

Kenneth D. Rothstein, MD serves on the Speakers Bureau for Three Rivers Pharmaceuticals, Roche, and Gilead, and serves on the Advisory Committee for Onny.

Jeffrey S. Sager, MD, MSc is an industry funded research/investigator for Actelion, is a consultant for Actelion, Gilead, and United Therapeutics, serves on the Speakers Bureau for Actelion and Gilead, and serves on the Advisory Board for Actelion.

Arun J. Sanyal, MBBS, MD is an industry funded research/investigator for Gilead Sciences, Inc., and Orphan Therapeutics, and serves on the Advisory Board for Ikaria and Salix.

David A. Sass, MD, FACP, FACG (Guest Editor) serves on the Speakers Bureau for Roche Pharmaceuticals and serves on the Advisory Committee for Gilead Sciences, Biotest Pharmaceuticals, and Bayer Healthcare pharmaceuticals.

Obaid S. Shaikh, MD, FRCP is an industry funded research/investigator for Ocera Therapeutics.

Disclosure of Discussion of Non-FDA Approved Uses for Pharmaceutical Products and/or Medical Devices.

The University of Virginia School of Medicine, as an ACCME provider, requires that all faculty presenters identify and disclose any off-label uses for pharmaceutical and medical device products. The University of Virginia School of Medicine recommends that each physician fully review all the available data on new products or procedures prior to clinical use.

TO ENROLL

To enroll in the Medical Clinics of North America Continuing Medical Education program, call customer service at 1-800-654-2452 or visit us online at http://www.theclinics.com/home/cme. The CME program is available to subscribers for an additional fee of USD 205.

THE CLINICS ARE NOW AVAILABLE ONLINE!

Access your subscription at:
www.theclinics.com

Contributors

GUEST EDITOR

DAVID A. SASS, MD
Associate Professor of Medicine and Surgery, Division of Gastroenterology and
Hepatology; Medical Director of Liver Transplantation, Drexel University College
of Medicine, Philadelphia, Pennsylvania

AUTHORS

JAWAD AHMAD, MD, MRCP
Associate Professor of Medicine, Division of Gastroenterology, Hepatology and Nutrition,
University of Pittsburgh School of Medicine, Pittsburgh, Pennsylvania

ZYGIMANTAS C. ALSAUSKAS, MD
Nephrology Fellow, Division of Nephrology, Department of Medicine, Mount Sinai School
of Medicine, New York, New York

KAPIL B. CHOPRA, MD, DM
Associate Professor of Medicine, Division of Gastroenterology, Hepatology and Nutrition,
University of Pittsburgh School of Medicine, Pittsburgh, Pennsylvania

MATTHEW COHEN, MD
Clinical Assistant Professor of Medicine, Department of Medicine, Drexel University
College of Medicine; Attending, Department of Gastroenterology, Frankford Hospital,
Philadelphia, Pennsylvania

JUAN F. GALLEGOS-OROZCO, MD
Gastroenterology Fellow, Division of Gastroenterology, Department of Medicine, Mayo
Clinic Arizona, Scottsdale, Arizona

WEI HOU, MD
Fellow, Division of Gastroenterology, Hepatology and Nutrition, Department of Internal
Medicine, Virginia Commonwealth University School of Medicine, Richmond, Virginia

HARVEY B. LEFTON, MD
Clinical Professor of Medicine, Department of Medicine, Drexel University College
of Medicine; Chief, Department of Gastroenterology, Frankford Hospital, Philadelphia,
Pennsylvania

LINA MACKELAITE, MD
Nephrology Fellow, Division of Nephrology, Department of Medicine, Drexel University
College of Medicine, Philadelphia, Pennsylvania

SHAHID M. MALIK, MD
Fellow, Division of Gastroenterology, Hepatology and Nutrition, University of Pittsburgh
School of Medicine, Pittsburgh, Pennsylvania

GAURAV MEHTA, MD
Fellow, Division of Gastroenterology and Hepatology, Department of Medicine, Drexel University College of Medicine, Philadelphia, Pennsylvania

MANUEL MENDIZABAL, MD
Staff Hepatologist, Servicio de Hepatología, Trasplante Hepático y Cirugía Hepatobiliar, Hospital Universitario Austral, Pilar, Argentina

KARTHIK RANGANNA, MD
Assistant Professor of Medicine, Division of Nephrology, Department of Medicine, Drexel University College of Medicine, Philadelphia, Pennsylvania

K. RAJENDER REDDY, MD
Professor of Medicine; Director of Hepatology; Medical Director of Liver Transplantation, Department of Medicine, University of Pennsylvania, Philadelphia, Pennsylvania

ANTHONY ROSA, MD
Clinical Assistant Professor of Medicine, Department of Medicine, Drexel University College of Medicine; Attending, Department of Gastroenterology, Frankford Hospital, Philadelphia, Pennsylvania

KENNETH D. ROTHSTEIN, MD
Associate Professor of Medicine; Chief, Division of Gastroenterology and Hepatology, Department of Medicine, Drexel University College of Medicine, Philadelphia, Pennsylvania

J.S. SAGER, MD, MSc
Medical Director, Cottage Pulmonary Hypertension Center; Clinical Assistant Professor, Department of Medicine, Keck School of Medicine, University of Southern California, Santa Barbara, California

ARUN J. SANYAL, MBBS, MD
Professor of Medicine, Division of Gastroenterology, Hepatology and Nutrition, Department of Internal Medicine, Virginia Commonwealth University School of Medicine, Richmond, Virginia

DAVID A. SASS, MD
Associate Professor of Medicine and Surgery, Division of Gastroenterology and Hepatology; Medical Director of Liver Transplantation, Drexel University College of Medicine, Philadelphia, Pennsylvania

OBAID S. SHAIKH, MD, FRCP
Associate Professor of Medicine, Division of Gastroenterology, Hepatology and Nutrition, University of Pittsburgh School of Medicine, Pittsburgh, Pennsylvania

C. SINGH, MD
Internal Medicine Resident, Santa Barbara Cottage Hospital, Buellton, California

VINAY SUNDARAM, MD
Fellow, Division of Gastroenterology, Hepatology and Nutrition, University of Pittsburgh School of Medicine, Pittsburgh, Pennsylvania

HUGO E. VARGAS, MD
Professor of Medicine, Division of Transplantation Medicine, Department of Medicine, Mayo Clinic Arizona, Phoenix, Arizona

Contents

Cirrhosis is defined histologically as an advanced form of progressive hepatic fibrosis with distortion of the hepatic architecture and regenerative nodule formation. It may be due to a variety of causes. It can be diagnosed incidentally on liver biopsy or hepatic imaging studies, or patients may present clinically with one or more features of hepatic failure. This article gives the reader a broad overview of the epidemiology, diagnosis, and natural history of cirrhosis; laying the foundation for subsequent articles, which will discuss the diagnosis and management of each of the specific cirrhosis-related complications.

Ascites is the pathologic accumulation of fluid in the peritoneal cavity and is a common manifestation of liver failure, being one of the cardinal signs of portal hypertension. The diagnostic evaluation of ascites involves an assessment of its cause by determining the serum-ascites albumin gradient and the exclusion of complications eg, spontaneous bacterial peritonitis. Although sodium restriction and diuretics remain the cornerstone of ascites management, many patients require additional therapy when they become refractory to such medical treatment. These include repeated large volume paracentesis and transjugular intrahepatic portosystemic shunts. This review article summarizes diagnostic tools and provides an evidence-based approach to the management of ascites.

Hepatic encephalopathy is characterized by neuropsychiatric abnormalities in patients with liver failure. Severe hepatic encephalopathy is an indication for liver transplantation as it portends poor outcome. Treatment of hepatic encephalopathy involves correction of precipitating factors such as sepsis, gastrointestinal bleeding, medications, and electrolyte imbalance. Effective therapies include lactulose and antibiotics such as neomycin, metronidazole, and rifaximin.

Portal hypertension is a progressively debilitating complication of cirrhosis and a principal cause of mortality in patients who have hepatic decompensation. This article describes the classification system and pathophysiology of portal hypertension. It also discusses a practical approach to prevention of first variceal hemorrhage, general management of the acute bleeding episode, and secondary prophylaxis to prevent rebleeding. Pharmacologic, endoscopic, radiologic, and surgical modalities are all described in detail.

modifications, and providing instructions on when to go to the emergency room (ER). There are also specific recommendations geared toward the patient with cirrhosis relating to slowing down the disease process, maintaining quality of life, and improving survival.

Patients with underlying liver disease often present for non–liver-related surgery and are at risk for postoperative decompensation. Several predictive models exist to determine the risk of morbidity and mortality after surgery in such patients, but the risk depends on the severity of liver disease and also the type and urgency of the surgery. Clinicians should be cognizant of the various risk assessment tools and incorporate them into their practice when encountering patients with liver disease undergoing surgery.

The widespread availability of transplantation in most major medical centers in the United States, together with a growing number of transplant candidates, has made it necessary for primary care providers, especially Internal Medicine and Family Practice physicians to be active in the clinical care of these patients before and after transplantation. This review provides an overview of the liver transplantation process, including indications, contraindications, time of referral to a transplant center, the current organ allocation system, and briefly touches on the expanding field of living donor liver transplantation.

Preface

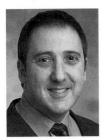

David A. Sass, MD
Guest Editor

Managing patients with cirrhosis and chronic liver failure can be a daunting task for the practicing clinician. Cirrhosis has become a very common disease as a result of the persistent high alcohol intake in many countries; the increased frequency of chronic hepatitis B and C infection; and the rising epidemic of obesity, the metabolic syndrome, and nonalcoholic steatohepatitis in the United States. Another factor emphasizing its importance as a disease entity is that cirrhosis and its complications are among the leading causes of death in many countries. In addition, the wide applicability and tremendous success of liver transplantation for hepatic failure has made this surgery a standard therapeutic procedure. For all of these reasons, it is timely to devote an issue of *Medical Clinics of North America* to "Care of the Cirrhotic Patient."

This issue presents a collection of 10 original review articles that cover the complete spectrum of inpatient and outpatient management of cirrhosis and its attendant complications. I am extremely privileged to have secured the participation of clinicians from multiple disciplines who are well-known experts in their respective areas. These articles are clinically oriented and are designed to provide internists with the necessary up-to-date, evidence-based information for optimal management of this complex group of patients. The reviews also emphasize the multidisciplinary approach that is required to effectively treat patients with decompensated liver disease.

First, Dr. Lefton and coauthors introduce the topic of cirrhosis by describing its clinical presentation and other epidemiologic aspects. Next, Dr. Sanyal and his colleague discuss the management of ascites by emphasizing its pathophysiology and also cover treatment options for refractory cases by large volume paracentesis and transjugular intrahepatic portosystemic shunt. Following this, Dr. Shaikh and his coauthor delve into the neurologic manifestations of liver failure by providing a comprehensive review of the topic of hepatic encephalopathy. Next, Drs. Sass and Chopra provide an overview of the management of varices, including primary and secondary prophylactic strategies and treatment of the acutely bleeding patient. Renal failure occurring in a cirrhotic patient may portend a very poor prognosis, especially that due to type 1 hepatorenal syndrome. Dr. Ranganna and colleagues discuss the differential diagnosis of kidney disease occurring in patients with advanced liver failure and

Med Clin N Am 93 (2009) xi–xii
doi:10.1016/j.mcna.2009.04.001
0025-7125/09/$ – see front matter

medical.theclinics.com

how such patients ought to be managed. Dr. Sager provides a comprehensive overview of an array of pulmonary manifestations of cirrhosis and the importance of screening for these complications, particularly during the liver transplant evaluation process. Dr. Reddy and coauthor next discuss the management options for cirrhotic patients who are diagnosed with hepatocellular carcinoma. They eloquently indicate the role of liver transplantation in such cases and highlight other locoregional therapies that may be used as a bridge to transplantation. The subsequent 2 articles review topics that are not frequently covered but are of particular relevance to the internist. Drs. Rothstein and Ahmad provide impressive reviews on preventative health issues and preoperative risk assessment in cirrhosis, respectively. Finally, to conclude this issue, Dr. Vargas and coauthor provide a comprehensive overview of liver transplantation and discuss the evolution of organ allocation from the Child-Pugh score to the MELD score.

I sincerely hope that this series of articles is informative and topical and provides useful tips to internists in managing this rather complex patient population. I truly appreciate all the effort put forth by the assembled panel of authors and their attention to detail in preparing their manuscripts for publication. I also thank Rachel Glover at Elsevier for her editorial assistance and guidance in the preparation of this issue.

David A. Sass, MD
Division of Gastroenterology and Hepatology
Drexel University College of Medicine
216 N. Broad Street, Feinstein Building, Suite 504
Philadelphia, PA 19102, USA

E-mail address:
dsass@drexelmed.edu (D.A. Sass)

Diagnosis and Epidemiology of Cirrhosis

Harvey B. Lefton, MD[a,b],*, Anthony Rosa, MD[a,b], Matthew Cohen, MD[a,b]

KEYWORDS

- Cirrhosis • Causes • Radiology • Labs • Clinical course

CIRRHOSIS: DIAGNOSIS AND EPIDEMIOLOGY

Cirrhosis is the end stage of chronic damage to the liver. It is characterized by fibrosis resulting in distortion and destruction of normal liver architecture. Functional liver tissue is destroyed and replaced by regenerating nodules that do not fully restore lost liver function. As the progressive cascade of liver tissue destruction continues, the patient shows signs of decreased mental, physical, and biochemical function. The final result of this relentless process is complete liver failure and death. The advent of liver transplantation has given the hope of returning to normal life to the patient with lost liver function.

Causes of Cirrhosis

Liver injury may be the result of infectious, autoimmune, vascular, hereditary, or chemical factors.

Viral hepatitis

Viral infection by hepatitis A is usually a nonfatal, self-limited disease characterized by a short period of disability followed by complete recovery.[1] Rarely will acute liver failure occur. In most cases, this illness is more a nuisance than a lethal process. When liver failure occurs in hepatitis A, it is usually submassive necrosis without cirrhosis, complete collapse of liver cells and architecture.

Similar to hepatitis A, hepatitis E is a self-limited process usually resulting in complete resolution of disease.[2] This virus does not contribute to cirrhosis but may manifest as an acute lethal form in pregnant patients in their third trimester.

[a] Department of Medicine, Drexel University College of Medicine, 216 Broad Street, Mail 1001, Philadelphia, PA 19102, USA
[b] Department of Gastroenterology, Frankford Hospital, 3998 Red Lion Road, Philadelphia, PA 19114, USA
* Corresponding author. Department of Gastroenterology, Frankford Hospital, 3998 Red Lion Road, Philadelphia, PA 19114.
E-mail address: hblmd@aol.com (H.B. Lefton).

Med Clin N Am 93 (2009) 787–799
doi:10.1016/j.mcna.2009.03.002
0025-7125/09/$ – see front matter © 2009 Elsevier Inc. All rights reserved.
medical.theclinics.com

Hepatitis B is a DNA virus, unlike the other common hepatotropic viruses, which are RNA viruses.[3] It may occur as a discrete entity or as part of a coinfection with hepatitis D, or delta infection. Although hepatitis B usually presents as a monoinfection, its presence is necessary for the delta virus to be infective. The hepatitis B virus may lead to chronic liver disease and cirrhosis. Hepatocellular carcinoma is a potential complication in these patients, even in the absence of cirrhosis. There is an increased incidence of this infection in Asia and sub-Saharan Africa.

Hepatitis C is an RNA virus that may cause chronic infection in 80% of patients and cirrhosis in 15% of patients.[4] The propensity to cirrhosis and liver cancer in patients with hepatitis C is increased in patients who are alcoholics. The advent of treatment with interferon and ribavirin has resulted in a halt in progression of disease and reversal of fibrosis and cirrhosis in some patients who respond to therapy.[5]

Vaccines are not available for patients with hepatitis D, C, or E; however, hepatitis A and B are vaccine-preventable infections.[6]

Alcohol

Alcohol is an important cause of liver disease and cirrhosis in the United States. Patients presenting for evaluation of abnormal liver function tests should be queried about their alcohol use. Cases of cirrhosis without any apparent cause should be investigated for alcohol use as the etiology. The ingestion of "tonics" was a cause of alcoholic liver disease in the early part of the last century, as these nostrums were often strongly fortified with alcohol. Today the "social drinker" must be challenged to determine the alcohol consumption, as most drinkers often underestimate or hide their consumption of alcohol. Heavy alcohol consumption may result in cirrhosis in 1 to 2 years or may be manifested several years after cessation of drinking. It is usual for alcoholic cirrhosis to occur after several years of heavy alcohol intake. Just as cigarette lung damage is measured in *pack years*, *pint years* can be used to measure alcohol damage, with 15 pint years being a reliable measure for cirrhosis (1 pt of whiskey per day for 15 years).[7] Heavier daily alcohol consumption would cause earlier cirrhosis. Concomitant infection with hepatitis C will accelerate cirrhosis formation in the alcoholic patient. The typical lesion seen on liver biopsy in alcoholics is the Mallory body, hyaline degeneration of the liver cell. This also may be seen in primary biliary cirrhosis,[8] Wilson disease,[9] and focal nodular hyperplasia[10] as large accumulations of eosinophilic material in the cytoplasm of hepatocytes.

Nonalcoholic fatty liver disease

There is an epidemic of obesity in children and adults in the United States. Many of these patients have nonalcoholic fatty liver disease (NAFLD). The spectrum of NAFLD includes nonalcoholic steatohepatitis, which can lead to fibrosis and cirrhosis. The only valued treatment available at present is weight reduction along with correction of lipid and glucose abnormalities. The growing numbers of patients with obesity seems to guarantee that more patients will progress to cirrhosis at an earlier age in the future.[11]

Autoimmune causes

Patients with autoimmune disorders are another source of chronic liver disease leading to cirrhosis. Primary biliary cirrhosis (PBC), a disorder that often affects middle-aged women, is characterized by cholestatic liver enzymes and positive anti-mitochondrial antibodies.[12] Patients typically develop progressive liver dysfunction resulting in cirrhosis and death if transplantation is not performed.

Primary sclerosing cholangitis (PSC) typically affects young men. It may occur up to 80% of the time with inflammatory bowel disease (especially ulcerative colitis) or as a primary entity.[13] There is no specific serologic marker, and diagnosis is usually made by noting a "pruned tree" deformity of bile ducts on endoscopic retrograde cholangio-pancreatography or magnetic resonance cholangiopancreatography.

Autoimmune hepatitis, an inflammatory condition of the liver, has unknown etiology and causes progressive liver dysfunction.[14] The presence of anti–smooth muscle anti-bodies, antinuclear antibodies, and increased serum gamma globulins help suggest the diagnosis. Other autoimmune disorders may also be present (Sjögren syndrome, thyroiditis, glomerulonephritis). Patients not responding to steroids and immune suppressive therapy may progress to cirrhosis.

Genetic disorder

The genetic diseases α_1-antitrypsin deficiency, Wilson disease, and hemochromatosis may be associated with cirrhosis. Because these diseases have a hereditary basis, all family members should be screened when a diagnosis is made in one family member. These diseases accounted for "cryptogenic cirrhosis" in the past. Cirrhotics with emphysema and children with cholestasis should be evaluated for α_1-antitrypsin defi-ciency.[15] Young patients who present with abnormal transaminases and have evidence of hemolysis and psychiatric and neurologic findings should be checked for elevated serum copper levels and low ceruloplasmin to exclude Wilson disease.[16] Diagnosis can be confirmed by checking a 24-hour urine copper test and a slit-lamp examination of the eye for Kayser-Fleischer rings. Prompt treatment with penicillamine or trientine will help reverse systemic effects of elevated serum copper and prevent liver failure in these patients.

Hereditary hemochromatosis, an inborn error of iron overload, may also result in liver, cardiac, pancreatic, and joint malfunction. These individuals usually present with a high serum ferritin and elevated iron saturation.[17] HFE mutation testing usually confirms C282Y homozygosity or compound heterozygosity with C282Y and H63D in most cases. Secondary iron overload with liver damage can occur in alcoholics, thal-assemia major, and patients who have required multiple transfusions, such as in sickle cell disease.

Rare causes

Some less common reported causes of cirrhosis are listed in **Box 1**; 10% to 15% of cases of cirrhosis remain "cryptogenic" when no etiology can be easily identified.

Clinical aspects

With progressive liver dysfunction, the clinical picture of cirrhosis becomes apparent. The clinician may first recognize cutaneous and scleral yellowing, which indicates the inability to clear bilirubin. Spider angiomas, collections of small vessels on the face, arms, and trunk, may be apparent. With the decreased synthesis of clotting factors produced by the liver, bruising and subcutaneous ecchymosis may be present. Low platelet counts can also lead to bleeding and bruising. Nail bed changes of paired hori-zontal white bands (Muehrcke nails) or nails with whitening of the proximal two thirds and reddening of the distal third (Terry nails) may be present. The patient may also have digital clubbing. One may find thickening of the palmar fascia (Dupuytren contracture) of the hands, especially in alcoholics.

Elevated estrogen levels can result in palmar erythema, gynecomastia, and testic-ular atrophy. This can also cause decreased libido and infertility.

When there is decreased clearing by the liver of mercaptans from the circulation, a sweet odor is noticeable in the breath of patients, the "fetor hepaticus." Also, parotid gland enlargement may occur. This painless swelling of the gland occurs in the absence of obstruction of the Stensen duct. Although not limited to end-stage liver

| **Box 1** |
| **Some miscellaneous causes of cirrhosis** |

Drugs

Oxyphenisatin

α-Methyldopa

Methotrexate

Amiodarone

Nitrofurantoin

Hypervitaminosis A

Metabolic errors

Glycogen storage diseases

Hereditary tyrosinemia

Mucopolysaccharoidosis

Infections

Syphilis

Schistosomiasis

Assorted entities

Sarcoidosis

Graft-versus-host disease

Budd-Chiari syndrome

Chronic congestive heart failure

Chronic ductal obstruction (secondary biliary cirrhosis)

Poisons

Carbon tetrachloride exposure

Dimethylnitrosamine exposure

disease, the flapping tremor of asterixis may be seen in patients with rising serum ammonia levels. Altered mentation and coma develop with progressive liver impairment and decreased toxin clearance by the dysfunctional liver.

Abdominal examination may demonstrate an enlarged, tender liver, but more often, the organ is difficult to palpate because of its fibrotic, shrunken state. This scarred organ diminishes blood flow resulting in increased back pressure in the portal system. Splenic enlargement may be present on abdominal examination. Blood flow can collateralize into the gastric and esophageal venous system causing gastric and esophageal varices. When pressure in the venous system reaches a critical level, rupture of these vessels can occur leading to life-threatening hematemesis (discussed further in another article). Back pressure in the portal circulation may cause colonic varices and hemorrhoids and "caput medusae" (portosystemic collaterals around the umbilicus). Late in cirrhosis, increased shunting of pressure into the splanchnic circulation will cause ascites, with fluid migrating into the abdomen, lower extremities, scrotum, or vulva. This condition is aggravated by hypoalbuminemia related to decreased hepatic protein synthesis. The risk of infection is also increased. The presence of ascites is associated with a shortened life expectancy with a 50% 2-year survival (see more on the natural history of ascites in another article).

RADIOLOGIC, BIOCHEMICAL, AND HISTOLOGIC FINDINGS OF CIRRHOSIS

Often, cirrhosis is diagnosed using a combination of clinical, radiographic, biochemical, and histologic findings. However, at times, the diagnosis may remain elusive despite a thorough noninvasive work-up because no single radiologic or biochemical test precisely correlates with a specific liver injury or degree of inflammation. Liver biopsy remains the only definitive marker of progression from chronic hepatitis to cirrhosis.[18]

Biochemical Markers of Cirrhosis

Because there is no single biochemical marker of cirrhosis, a biochemical work-up with conventional liver function tests (LFTs) is often initiated when clinical symptoms are identified or when stigmata of chronic liver disease are apparent on physical examination. Liver function panels commonly include alanine aminotransferase (ALT), aspartate aminotransferase (AST), bilirubin, alkaline phosphatase, prothrombin time (PT), and albumin. Interpretation of LFTs and the decision to initiate further testing must be made in the context of the history and physical examination.

The AST, ALT, bilirubin, and alkaline phosphatase are not true indicators of hepatic function. AST and ALT are hepatic enzymes that are released into the bloodstream from damaged hepatocytes after hepatocellular injury or death. ALT is considered to be a cost-effective screening test for hepatic inflammation. It is useful in narrowing the differential diagnosis in acute and chronic liver injury. It serves a limited role in predicting the degree of liver inflammation but no role in predicting the severity of fibrosis.[18,19] Several studies have demonstrated a significant overlap in ALT levels among mild, moderate, and severe histologic activity in patients with hepatitis C.[20,21]

The AST/ALT ratio has been investigated to help determine the degree of hepatic fibrosis in several studies.[22,23] The AST/ALT ratio is approximately 0.8 in normal subjects. In patients with alcoholic hepatitis, the ratio is frequently greater than 2:1.[24] In patients with nonalcoholic hepatitis, the ratio is typically less than 1 and increases to greater than 1 with an increasing fibrosis score.[23] In these studies, AST/ALT greater than 1 had a specificity of greater than 75% and sensitivity of 32% to 83% for cirrhosis.[22,23,25] However, 2 additional studies failed to corroborate the predictive value of the AST/ALT ratio, and therefore the clinical utility of this ratio remains unclear.[26,27]

The PT and serum albumin are more accurate markers of true hepatic synthetic function. Hepatic synthesis of clotting cascade proteins is required to maintain a normal prothrombin time. As the ability of the cirrhotic liver to synthesize clotting proteins diminishes, the prothrombin time increases. The PT helps predict survival probability in cirrhosis when used as a parameter in the Child-Pugh classification or model for end-stage liver disease (MELD) score. In one study among patients with alcoholic liver disease, the PT accurately and consistently correlated with the degree of liver fibrosis.[28] However, the PT is not specific for hepatic dysfunction; other disorders such as inherited coagulopathies, malabsorption, and malnutrition can account for abnormal clotting times.

Since albumin is synthesized exclusively in the liver, levels may decrease as synthetic function of the liver declines in cirrhosis. Similar to the PT, serum albumin levels have been used to predict prognosis in the Child-Pugh classification. Serum levels are affected by noncirrhotic conditions such as intestinal malabsorption, malnutrition, and nephrosis.

Thrombocytopenia, defined as a platelet count less than 150,000, is a common finding in patients with chronic liver disease. Moderate thrombocytopenia (platelet count, 50,000–75,000) can be found in approximately 13% of patients with cirrhosis.[29] Thrombocytopenia has been typically attributed to passive sequestration of platelets in the spleen. However, recent research suggests that decreased platelet production, increased destruction, and functional platelet disorders may contribute to thrombocytopenia in cirrhotic patients. A platelet count of 160,000 or less, although not used as an independent predictor of cirrhosis, was shown in 1 study to have a sensitivity of 80% and a specificity of 58% in detecting cirrhosis among patients with chronic hepatitis C.[30]

Various combinations of biochemical markers have been used to increase the accuracy in predicting cirrhosis and include the prothrombin time, gamma-glutamyl transpeptidase activity, and serum apolipoprotein A1 concentration (PGA) index, FIB-4, and FibroTest. The PGA ranges in accuracy between 66% and 72% for predicting cirrhosis in alcoholic patients.[31] The FIB-4 includes the AST, ALT, platelet count, and age and has a positive predictive value of 82% and specificity of 98% in predicting significant fibrosis in patients with hepatitis C.[32] The FibroTest includes α_2-macroglobulin, haptoglobin, gamma globulin, apolipoprotein A1, GGT, and total bilirubin. It has a sensitivity and specificity of 75% and 85%, respectively, for detecting severe fibrosis.[33]

The progressive course of fibrosis results in changes to the extracellular matrix of the hepatic parenchyma. Products of collagen synthesis, enzymes, cytokines, and chemokines involved in fibrogenesis have shown promise as direct markers of liver fibrosis. Examples include procollagen peptide, type IV collagen, laminin, hyaluronic acid, transforming growth factor beta, and matrix metalloproteinase. Although progress has been made in using these tests as direct, noninvasive markers of cirrhosis, their use does not eliminate the need for direct liver analysis by way of biopsy.

Once a diagnosis of cirrhosis is established, specific causes such as viral hepatitis, primary biliary cirrhosis, autoimmune hepatitis, Wilson disease, hemochromatosis, and α_1-antitrypsin deficiency are supported by the presence of certain serologic and biochemical markers (**Table 1**).

Radiologic Findings in Cirrhosis

No specific radiologic test can establish a diagnosis of cirrhosis. Abdominal ultrasound, CT, and MRI are most useful for supporting the clinical or histologic diagnosis of cirrhosis by identifying manifestations such as hepatomegaly, splenomegaly, hepatic nodularity, ascites, portal vein thrombosis (PVT), portal hypertension, portosystemic collateral vessels (varices), and hepatocellular carcinoma (HCC).

Abdominal ultrasound is typically the first imaging modality used to evaluate cirrhosis. It is comparatively inexpensive and poses no risk of contrast or radiation exposure to the patient. Cirrhosis is characterized by a coarsened, heterogeneous echo pattern with surface nodularity on ultrasound. The liver may appear atrophic in advanced disease. Caudate lobe hypertrophy is a common finding in cirrhosis. In one study, a sonographic ratio of caudate lobe width to right lobe width of 0.65 or greater yielded a sensitivity and specificity for cirrhosis of 84% and 100%, respectively.[34] Sonographic findings of portal hypertension include splenomegaly, ascites, and portosystemic collateral vessels. Furthermore, when conventional ultrasound is combined with Doppler sonography, thrombosis of the portal and hepatic veins can be identified, as can dilation of the superior mesenteric vein, portal vein, and hepatic artery. Hepatofugal portal flow, the reversal of normal portal flow toward the liver, can be detected with color Doppler ultrasound.

In general, hepatic ultrasound is not reliable in detecting hepatocellular carcinoma. Significant variability exists in the sonographic appearance of prominent regenerative

Table 1
Biochemical and histologic markers of various causes of cirrhosis

Etiology	Biochemical Markers	Characteristic Histologic Findings
Alcoholic liver disease	AST/ALT >2 Elevated GGT	Mallory bodies Giant mitochondria Centrilobular fibrosis Ballooned hepatocytes
α_1-Antitrypsin deficiency	Decreased α_1-antitrypsin Pi type ZZ or SZ	Eosinophilic globules in periportal zones Periodic acid–Schiff deposits

Autoimmune hepatitis	Positive ANA titer
	Positive ASMA titer
	Positive LKM Ab
	Elevated globulins
	  (especially serum IgG)
		Lymphoid aggregates
		Prominent plasma cells
		Interface hepatitis
		Rosetting of hepatocytes
		  (Duct damage)

Hepatitis B	Positive HbsAg ± eAg
	  positivity
	Positive HepB DNA
	Elevated ALT, AST
		Ground glass cells containing
		  HBsAg

Hepatitis C	Positive HCV Ab Positive HCV RNA Elevated ALT, AST	Bile duct damage Lymphocyte infiltration

Hereditary hemochromatosis	Fasting transferrin
	  saturation >45%
	Elevated ferritin
	HFE gene mutation
		Iron deposition within
		  hepatocytes

Primary biliary cirrhosis	Positive AMA Elevated serum IgM	Loss of interlobular ducts Ductal inflammation "Florid duct" lesion Granulomas
Primary sclerosing cholangitis	Elevated p-ANCA	Bile duct scarring Concentric ("onion-skin") fibrosis
Wilson disease	Ceruloplasmin <20 24-h urinary copper excretion >100 mcg	Copper deposits Focal, may be missed on biopsy Mallory bodies

nodules, dysplastic nodules, and hepatocellular carcinoma. Therefore, the detection of hepatic nodules on ultrasound always warrants further diagnostic cross-sectional imaging with CT or MRI.

Parenchymal distortion caused by cirrhosis produces characteristic changes easily recognized on contrast-enhanced CT and MRI. Typically these changes include a nodular liver margin, atrophy, hypertrophy, and heterogeneity induced by fibrosis, steatosis, and iron deposition. The radiologic changes become easier to identify as cirrhosis progresses to advanced disease.

Distinguishing regenerative nodules from dysplastic nodules and HCC is challenging with contrast-enhanced CT and MRI. On MRI regenerative nodules may appear hypointense on T2-weighted images and isointense on T1-weighted images, but this is not always the rule. Dysplastic lesions can go completely undetected on MRI and CT.[35] Arterial phase CT scans can detect HCC by demonstrating characteristic arterioportal shunting within a hepatic mass, although this pattern can be seen in cirrhotic livers without tumor.[36] Although portal venous phase CT and magnetic resonance angiography can detect portal vein thrombosis and flow, these studies are expensive, and routine ultrasound with Doppler is often adequate to obtain the same information. For these reasons, CT and MRI may be best used as follow-up tests to assess interval changes in size and appearance of known hepatic lesions.

Histologic Patterns of Cirrhosis

Liver biopsy is the gold standard for establishing the diagnosis of cirrhosis. The sensitivity and specificity for diagnosing cirrhosis by liver biopsy range from 80% to 100% and are dependent upon the number and size of samples. Biopsy also serves to grade and stage the severity of fibrosis and thus provides important information for management and prognosis. However, percutaneous transabdominal liver biopsy has potential risks. Foremost, it is an invasive procedure and may result in perforated viscera, bleeding, and infection. Additionally, biopsy specimens are prone to sampling error since only a small segment of liver parenchyma is obtained.

Certain pathologic features are common to all forms of cirrhosis and include hepatic parenchymal necrosis, replacement of normal parenchyma with nodular regeneration, and connective tissue deposition resulting in scarring.[36] Various causes of liver disease have characteristic histopathologic findings, and the more common causes will be reviewed here.

Grossly, cirrhosis can be classified as micronodular, macronodular, or mixed.

Alcoholic liver disease is generally described as micronodular cirrhosis; the liver surface is irregular and diffusely covered with small regenerative nodules of uniform size, measuring on average less than 3 mm in diameter.[36] Grossly, the liver is enlarged, measuring 1500 to 2000 g, but as cirrhosis progresses, the liver shrinks in size and nodules become larger. Microscopically, Mallory bodies and diffuse fat accumulation are frequently present. Though commonly found in alcoholic liver disease, they are not specific and may be seen in other causes of cirrhosis. Steatosis is generally macroscopic wherein large fat droplets displace the nuclei to the periphery of the hepatocyte. Fat accumulation, most prominent in the pericentral (centrilobular) zone, can progress to complete obliteration of the central vein. The pattern is described as a "central-central" pattern of cirrhosis where portal zones are connected by thin bands of connective tissue. This gives a characteristic "chicken-wire" appearance on trichrome stain. Giant mitochondria and collagenization of the space of Disse can be seen on electron microscopy.

Chronic viral hepatitis is the most common cause of macronodular cirrhosis. Grossly, this pattern of liver injury is characterized by a dense, shrunken liver, with large regenerative nodules connected by broad bands of connective tissue. Microscopically, irregular bands of connective tissue are prominent and will often encompass three or more portal tracts in a single scar. In hepatitis B, the "ground glass hepatocyte" containing HBsAg may be identified on hematoxylin and eosin stain. Bile duct damage and lymphocyte infiltration may be more prominent in cirrhosis caused by hepatitis C.

Cardiac cirrhosis can result from chronic congestive heart failure or constrictive pericarditis and typically resembles alcoholic cirrhosis. Grossly, the liver is nodular, and microscopically there is centrilobular sclerosis. However, the hallmark of cardiac cirrhosis is the presence of dilated, blood filled hepatic sinusoids.[37] Erythrocyte breakdown results in accumulation of hemosiderin and lipid laden macrophages. The fibrous deposition bridges central areas with relative portal sparing. Cirrhosis caused by venous outflow obstruction or Budd-Chiari syndrome results from obstruction of the hepatic vein. This can present as a central pattern similar to cardiac cirrhosis, with sinusoidal congestion and hepatic necrosis.

Biliary cirrhosis caused by PBC or PSC manifests in a broad spectrum of histologic findings but always involves the bile ducts. Typical histologic findings that distinguish biliary cirrhosis from other causes include loss of interlobular bile ducts and ductal inflammation.[37] Portal tract damage results in a characteristic portal-portal fibrosis or "jigsaw" pattern of cirrhosis microscopically. Chronic inflammation around cholangioles and disruption of the terminal plate results in interface hepatitis, previously known as biliary piecemeal necrosis.[37] Copper is often deposited and may be seen with orcein stain. In contrast to other patterns of cirrhosis, central veins are rarely involved or become involved late in disease progression.

Distinguishing PBC from PSC can be difficult with liver biopsy early in the course but becomes easier with disease progression. In general, an increased mononuclear infiltrate in the sinusoids, portal-based granulomas, and hepatocyte necrosis are typical histologic features of PBC. Ductal scarring and periductal fibrosis of both large and small ducts is a classic finding in PSC.[37]

The hallmark histologic findings of other causes of cirrhosis are summarized in **Table 1**.

PROGRESSION FROM COMPENSATED TO DECOMPENSATED CIRRHOSIS

The onset of complications related to cirrhosis occurs in the setting of worsening portal hypertension and hepatic insufficiency and defines the transition from a compensated state to decompensation. These complications, which negatively impact the quality of life and prognosis of the cirrhotic patient, include ascites, jaundice, variceal hemorrhage, and portosystemic encephalopathy. Other complications such as spontaneous bacterial peritonitis, hepatic hydrothorax, hepatorenal syndrome, portopulmonary hypertension, HCC, and PVT may accelerate clinical deterioration. Hepatic decompensation develops at an advanced stage of cirrhosis that is generally considered to be irreversible. Although hepatic fibrogenesis has been demonstrated to be a dynamic and potentially reversible process, the point at which advanced fibrosis or cirrhosis becomes irreversible is yet to be identified.[38] Slowing or reversing the progression of chronic liver disease before decompensation by addressing the specific causes of hepatocellular injury may improve the high morbidity and mortality of cirrhosis. Cirrhotic patients should be monitored for the development of the complications of end-stage liver disease. When they arise, directed therapies should be undertaken to address these often devastating clinical events. In many instances, the onset of hepatic decompensation serves as a clinical cue to initiate evaluation for liver transplantation in appropriate patients.

The natural history of cirrhosis is typically characterized by a prolonged asymptomatic phase of compensated disease. The median survival from the time of diagnosis of compensated cirrhosis is 10 to 12 years.[39,40] During this period, patients should be monitored for the development of complications and hepatic insufficiency, which includes interval screening for gastroesophageal varices and HCC. Furthermore, patients should be advised to avoid any potentially hepatoxic agents and susceptible patients should be vaccinated against hepatitis A and hepatitis B to decrease the risk of superimposed hepatic insult.[41] Progression to decompensated disease has been estimated to occur in approximately 60% of cirrhotic patients at 10 years after diagnosis.[39] However, the likelihood of decompensation for individual patients is highly variable and can be difficult to predict. This is due to factors that include the etiology of cirrhosis, the ability to eliminate or treat the cause(s) of chronic liver disease, preserved hepatic synthetic function or hepatic reserve, existing comorbidities, and the development of infection and HCC. The ability to eliminate or treat the source of chronic liver disease is of particular importance in delaying decompensation and prolonging survival. Abstinence from alcohol has been demonstrated to improve survival in alcoholic cirrhotics.[42] The initiation of interferon therapy for patients with compensated HCV-related cirrhosis and antiviral therapy for patients with HBV-related cirrhosis may retard the progression of cirrhosis and decrease the risk of HCC.[43,44]

Decompensation develops when disease progression results in worsening portal hypertension and decreased hepatic reserve. The rate of decompensation is approximately 5% to 7% annually.[45] Once this transition occurs there is a marked reduction in life expectancy that is due, in large part, directly to the listed life-threatening complications. Upon decompensation, median survival time plummets to approximately 2 years.[39,40] Ascites is usually the first and most common sign of decompensation.[39] From the onset of ascites, the 2-year mortality is approximately 50%.[40] A staging system of the natural history of cirrhosis was agreed upon at the Baveno IV International Consensus Workshop. Each of the four stages is defined by the presence or absence of ascites, gastroesophageal varices, and variceal hemorrhage. The progression through each clinical stage is accompanied by a dramatic increase in mortality (**Fig. 1**). Stage 1, defined by the absence of varices and ascites, has a 1-year probability of death of 1%. The development of nonbleeding varices characterizes Stage 2, which carries a 1-year probability of death of 3.4%. Stage 3, the onset of decompensated cirrhosis, is defined as the development of ascites irrespective of the presence or absence of nonbleeding varices. The 1-year mortality is 20%. Stage 4, the development of variceal bleeding with or without ascites, has a 1-year mortality of 57%. Almost half of these deaths occur as the result of the initial bleeding episode.[45,46]

Although the course of cirrhosis is highly variable due to the influence of numerous factors, several prognostic models and scoring systems are used to stratify disease severity and predict survival. The Child-Pugh score, which incorporates five variables (bilirubin, albumin, PT, ascites, and encephalopathy), has been demonstrated to be a predictor of the development of cirrhosis-related complications and of survival.[47] The MELD score, calculated using bilirubin, international normalized ratio , and creatinine, was initially designed to predict the mortality of cirrhotic patients undergoing transjugular intrahepatic portosystemic shunt placement.[48] It is now used to prioritize patients awaiting organ allocation and has proved to be a predictor of survival. The Child-Pugh and MELD scores are discussed in greater detail elsewhere in this issue.

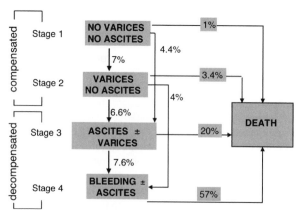

Fig.1. 1-year outcome probabilities according to clinical stage. (*From* D'Amico G, Garcia-Tsao G, Pagliaro L. Natural history and prognostic indicators of survival in cirrhosis: a systematic review of 118 studies. J Hepatol 2006;44:219; with permission.)

To summarize, although staging systems and models can provide useful prognostic information and risk stratification for a population of cirrhotic patients, a predictive assessment of decompensation and mortality for the individual patient may be challenging. When possible, the underlying cause of chronic liver disease should be addressed and treated. Additional hepatic insult should be minimized by the avoidance of hepatotoxic agents. When appropriate, vaccination against hepatitis A and hepatitis B is recommended. Regular assessments of hepatic synthetic function can detect a decline in hepatic reserve. Screening protocols for the development of gastroesophageal varices and HCC should be followed. After the development of varices, primary prophylaxis of variceal hemorrhage should be undertaken. With the onset of cirrhosis-related complications, early detection and an expeditious delivery of directed therapy improve patient survival and often serve as a bridge for eventual liver transplantation. Ultimately, greater understanding of the mechanisms of fibrosis development and reversibility may result in the emergence of future therapies that can alter the natural course of cirrhosis.

REFERENCES

1. Wasley A, Fiore A, Bell BP. Hepatitis A in the era of vaccination. Epidemiol Rev 2006;28:101–11.
2. Purcell RH, Emerson SU. Hepatitis E: an emerging awareness of an old disease. J Hepatol 2008;48(3):494–503.
3. Lok AS, McMahon BJ. Chronic hepatitis B. Hepatology 2007;45(2):507–39.
4. Leandro G, Mangia A, Hui J. Relationship between steatosis, inflammation, and fibrosis in chronic hepatitis C; a meta-analysis of individual patient data. Gastroenterology 2006;130:1636–42.
5. Poynard T, McHutchison J, Manns M, et al. Impact of pegylated interferon alfa-2b and ribavirin on liver fibrosis in patients with chronic hepatitis C. Gastroenterology 2002;122(5):1303–13.
6. Conjeevaram H. Viral hepatitis. AGA focused clinical updates 2005:195–204.
7. Conn H. Alcohol content of various beverages: all booze is created equal. Hepatology 1990;12:1252–8.
8. Fickert P, Trauner M, Fuchsbichler A, et al. Mallory body formation in primary biliary cirrhosis is associated with increased amounts and abnormal phosphorylation and ubiquitination of cytokeratins. J Hepatol 2003;38(4):387–94.
9. French S. Mallory bodies, like the mutant ATP7B seen in Wilson disease, are aggresomes. Gastroenterology 2001;121(5):1264–6.
10. Agaimy A, Kaiser A, Wuensch PH. Severe cytological atypia (large cell change) in focal nodular hyperplasia with numerous mallory bodies. A benign (adaptive) change? Pathol Res Pract 2003;199(7):509–11.
11. Charlton M. Non-alcoholic fatty liver disease: a review of current understanding and future impact. Clin Gastroenterol Hepatol 2004;2:1048–58.
12. Kumagi T, Heathcote EJ. Primary biliary cirrhosis. Orphanet J Rare Dis 2008;3:1–17.
13. Lindor KD. Characteristics of primary sclerosing cholangitis in the USA. Hepatol Res 2007;37(Suppl 3):S474–7.
14. Czaja AJ. Autoimmune liver disease. Curr Opin Gastroenterol 2008;24(3):298–305.
15. Perlmutter DH. Alpha-1-antitrypsin deficiency: diagnosis and treatment. Clin Liver Dis 2004;8(4):839–59.

16. Roberts EA, Schilsky ML. Diagnosis and treatment of Wilson disease: an update. Hepatology 2008;47(6):2089–111.
17. Adams PC, Barton JC. Hemochromatosis. Lancet 2007;370(9602):1855–60.
18. Dufour D, Lott J, Nolte F, et al. Diagnosis and monitoring of hepatic injury. II. Recommendations for use of laboratory tests in screening, diagnosis, and monitoring. Clin Chem 2000;46:2050–68.
19. Heidelbaugh J, Bruderly M. Cirrhosis and chronic liver failure: part 1. Diagnosis and Evaluation. Am Fam Physician 2006;74:756–62.
20. Haber M, West A, Haber A, et al. Relationship of amiotransferases to liver histological status in chronic hepatitis C. Am J Gastroenterol 1995;90:1250–7.
21. Healey C, Chapman R, Fleming K. Liver histology in hepatitis C infection: a comparison between patients with persistently normal or abnormal transaminases. Gut 1995;37:274–8.
22. Bonacini M, Hadi G, Govindarajan S, et al. Utility of a discriminant score for diagnosing advanced fibrosis or cirrhosis in patients with chronic hepatitis C virus infection. Am J Gastroenterol 1997;92:1302–4.
23. Sheth S, Glamm S, Gordon F, et al. AST/ALT ratio predicts cirrhosis in patients with chronic hepatitis C virus infection. Am J Gastroenterol 1998;93:44–8.
24. Cohen J, Kaplan M. The SGOT/SGPT ratio—an indicator of alcoholic liver disease. Dig Dis Sci 1979;24(11):835–8.
25. Williams A, Hoofnagle J. Relationship of serum aspartate to alanine aminotransferase in chronic hepatitis. Relationship to cirrhosis. Gastroenterology 1988;95:734–9.
26. Imperiale T, Said A, Cummings O, et al. Need for validation of clinical decision aids: use of the AST/ALT ratio in predicting cirrhosis in chronic hepatitis C. Am J Gastroenterol 2000;95(9):2328–32.
27. Reedy D, Loo A, Levine R. AST/ALT ratio ≥1 is not diagnostic of cirrhosis in patients with chronic hepatitis C. Dig Dis Sci 1998;43(9):2156–9.
28. Croquet V, Vuillemin E, Ternisien C, et al. Prothrombin index is an indirect marker of severe liver fibrosis. Eur J Gastroenterol Hepatol 2002;14(10):1133–41.
29. Afdhal N, McHutchinson J, Brown R, et al. Thrombocytopenia associated with chronic liver disease. J Hepatol 2008;48(6):1000–7.
30. Pilette C, Oberte F, Aube C, et al. Non-invasive diagnosis of esophageal varices in chronic liver diseases. J Hepatol 1999;31(5):867–73.
31. Lu LG, Zeng MD, Mao YM, et al. Relationship between clinical and pathologic findings in patients with chronic liver diseases. World J Gastroenterol 2003;9(12):2796–800.
32. Vallet-Pichard A, Mallet V, Nalpas B, et al. FIB-4: an inexpensive and accurate marker of fibrosis in HCV infection. Comparison with liver biopsy and fibrotest. Hepatology 2007;46(1):32–6.
33. Rossi E, Adams L, Prins A, et al. Validation of the FibroTest biochemical markers score in assessing liver fibrosis in hepatitis C patients. Clin Chem 2003;49(3):450–4.
34. Harbin W, Robert N, Ferrucci J. Diagnosis of cirrhosis based on regional changes in hepatic morphology: a radiological and pathological analysis. Radiology 1980;135(2):273–83.
35. Gupta A, Kim D, Krinsky G, et al. CT and MRI of cirrhosis and its mimics. AJR Am J Roentgenol 2004;183:1595–601.
36. Brown J, Naylor M, Yagan N. Imaging of hepatic cirrhosis. Radiology 1997;202:1–16.
37. Ferrell L. Liver pathology: cirrhosis, hepatitis, and primary liver tumors. Update and diagnostic problems. Mod Pathol 2000;13(6):679–704.

38. Bonis P, Friedman S, Kaplan M. Is liver fibrosis reversible? N Engl J Med 2001; 344:452–4.
39. Gines P, Quintero E, Arroyo V. Compensated cirrhosis: natural history and prognostic factors. Hepatology 1987;7:122–8.
40. D'Amico G, Morabito A, Pagliaro L, et al. Survival and prognostic indicators in compensated and decompensated cirrhosis. Dig Dis Sci 1986;31:468–75.
41. National Institutes of Health Consensus Development Conference Panel Statement: Management of Hepatitis C 2002. Hepatology 2002;36(Suppl 1):S3–21.
42. Borowsky SA, Strome S, Lott E. Continued heavy drinking and survival in alcoholic cirrhosis. Gastroenterology 1981;80:1405–9.
43. Bruno S, Stroffolini T, Colombo M. Sustained virological response to interferon-alpha is associated with improved outcome in HCV-related cirrhosis: a retrospective study. Hepatology 2007;45:579–87.
44. Benvegnu L, Chemello L, Noventa F. Retrospective analysis of the effect of interferon therapy on the clinical outcome of patients with viral cirrhosis. Cancer 1998; 83:901–9.
45. D'Amico G, Garcia-Tsao G, Pagliaro L. Natural history and prognostic indicators of survival in cirrhosis: a systemic review of 118 studies. J Hepatol 2006;44: 217–31.
46. deFranchis R. Evolving consensus in portal hypertension. Report of the Baveno IV consensus workshop on methadology of diagnosis and therapy in portal hypertension. J Hepatol 2005;43(1):167–76.
47. Infante-Rivard C, Esnaola S, Villeneuve J. Clinical and statistical validity of conventional prognostic factors in predicting short-term survival among cirrhotics. Hepatology 1987;7(4):660–4.
48. Salerno F, Merli M, Cazzaniga M, et al. MELD score is better than Child-Pugh score in predicting 3-month survival of patients undergoing transjugular intrahepatic portosystemic shunt. J Hepatol 2002;36(4):494–500.

Ascites: Diagnosis and Management

Wei Hou, MD, Arun J. Sanyal, MBBS, MD*

KEYWORDS

- Cirrhosis • Ascites • Portal hypertension • Refractory ascites
- Transjugular intrahepatic portosystemic shunts
- Spironolactone • Furosemide
- Spontaneous bacterial peritonitis

Ascites is a common complication of cirrhosis. The development of ascites marks the onset of worsened prognosis and increased mortality in patients with cirrhosis. Ascites also causes considerable morbidity in the affected individual by producing abdominal distension, respiratory distress, formation of hernias especially around the umbilicus, worsening nutritional status, and increased susceptibility to infections. All of these contribute to repeated hospitalizations in such patients and markedly impair their quality of life. Appropriate management of ascites is thus an important pillar in the care of a patient with cirrhosis. The current concepts about the pathophysiology, diagnosis, and management of ascites are reviewed in the following sections.

PATHOPHYSIOLOGY

The main factor contributing to the development of ascites in a patient with cirrhosis is the portal hypertension which results from increased intrahepatic resistance to blood flow and is compounded by splanchnic vasodilatation as a result of local production of vasodilators (**Fig. 1**).[1–8] Cirrhosis occurs as a consequence of chronic liver injury–induced distortion of hepatic architecture and fibrosis. Increased resistance to portal blood flow as a result of cirrhosis and vascular tone because of increased production of vasoconstrictors, such as angiotensin, endothelin, cysteinyl-leukotrienes, and thromboxane leads to gradual formation of portal hypertension, collateral vein circulation, and shunting of blood to the systemic circulation. Splanchnic vasodilatation develops as persistent portal hypertension results in local overproduction of vasodilators such as nitric oxide (NO), calcitonin gene–related peptide, substance P, carbon monoxide, and endogenous cannabinoids. Among these vasodilators, NO is a potent

This work is original and not under consideration elsewhere for publication. It was supported in part by a grant from the NIH K24 DK 02755-09 to Dr. Sanyal.
Division of Gastroenterology, Hepatology and Nutrition, Department of Internal Medicine, Virginia Commonwealth University School of Medicine, MCV Box 980341, Richmond, VA 23298-0341, USA
* Corresponding author.
E-mail address: asanyal@mcvh-vcu.edu (A.J. Sanyal).

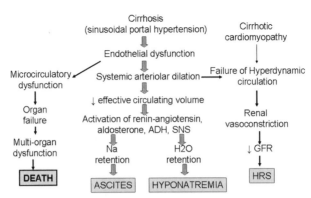

Fig. 1. The pathophysiology of cirrhosis and ascites is shown. Cirrhosis is associated with splanchnic arterial vasodilation. This leads to a decrease in effective circulating volume and a hyperdynamic circulation. The decrease in effective circulating volume causes activation of renal sodium and water retentive pathways (eg, RAAS, renal SNS, and ADH). The resulting sodium and water retention leads to ascites as a result of spillage of excess sodium and water from hepatic lymph into the peritoneal cavity. As the disease progresses, a progressive decrease in effective circulating volume develops, causing severe renal vasoconstriction and a decrease in glomerular filtration rate. The onset of cirrhotic cardiomyopathy accentuates this problem and tips the patient into hepatorenal syndrome. The accompanying circulatory disturbance leads to organ failure and death. Sepsis is frequently associated with this process.

and predominant vasodilator. Endothelial stretching and bacterial translocation are responsible for the local overproduction of vasodilators and other cytokines.[9,10] Recent data suggest that bacteria translocate to mesenteric lymph nodes in cirrhosis, and consequently stimulation of cytokine production plays an important role in the process of arterial vasodilatation.[11–13]

Splanchnic arteriolar vasodilation and consequent pooling of blood in the splanchnic circulation causes a decrease in effective arterial blood volume and arterial pressure. In response to this change in effective arterial blood volume and arterial pressure, baroreceptor-mediated activation of the sympathetic nervous system (SNS), renin-angiotensin-aldosterone system (RAAS), and antidiuretic hormone (ADH) cause avid renal water and sodium retention in order to restore homeostasis. Cirrhosis is also associated with increased sinusoidal pressure and decreased plasma oncotic pressure. These combine to increase hepatic lymph formation. When the capacity of the hepatic lymphatics to return hepatic lymph to the circulation is exceeded, the excess lymph (composed of an ultrafiltrate of plasma containing the retained sodium and water) spills into the peritoneal cavity, producing ascites.

The cardiac output and plasma volume increase in the early stages of liver cirrhosis, which maintains circulatory function compensated. However, decrease in cardiac output as a result of cirrhotic cardiomyopathy occurs in the advanced stage of liver cirrhosis and contributes to a further fall in effective arterial blood volume and arterial pressure. This causes marked activation of systemic vasoconstrictive mechanisms that particularly affect the kidneys and decrease glomerular filtration and renal plasma flow. In its most severe form, this leads to progressive renal failure, that is, hepatorenal syndrome.

DIAGNOSIS

The goals of the diagnostic assessment of a patient with ascites are to establish the presence of ascites, determine its severity, determine its cause, and detect the presence of complications of ascites, which include spontaneous bacterial peritonitis and renal failure. A good clinical assessment provides invaluable information about these goals.

A correct diagnosis of the cause of ascites is the essential first step to its successful treatment. Cirrhosis accounts for approximately 85% of ascites in the United States, whereas nonhepatic diseases cause most of the remaining cases (**Box 1**).[14] A history of risk factors for liver diseases such as viral hepatitis, alcohol abuse, metabolic syndrome, familial liver diseases, autoimmune disease, and so on should be obtained. Cancer is the second most common cause of ascites. A history of cancer should lead to exploring the possibility that ascites could be caused by peritoneal carcinomatosis. Heart failure is the third common cause of ascites and a history of heart failure could hint at a cardiogenic etiology as a potential cause of ascites. A history of tuberculosis, kidney disease on dialysis, pancreatic disease, and so on are also relevant, and questions about these less common diseases should also be asked.

The physical examination should focus on stigmata of cirrhosis and signs suggesting the presence of ascites. Stigmata of cirrhosis such as spider angioma and palmar erythema may coexist with ascites. A full and bulging abdomen should lead to the evaluation of ascites. Flank dullness on percussion is usually characteristic of ascites. A positive shifting dullness usually suggests the presence of more than 1500 mL of

---

Box 1
Causes of ascites

1. Portal hypertension

   Presinusoidal causes, eg, portal vein thrombosis (usually ascites is mild if present at all)

   Sinusoidal causes, eg, cirrhosis, vitamin A toxicity

   Postsinusoidal causes, eg, venoocclusive disease, Budd-Chiari syndrome, constrictive pericarditis, congestive heart failure

2. Neoplastic causes

   Peritoneal carcinomatosis

   Lymphoma

   Hepatocellular cancer

   Ovarian cancer

   Mesothelioma

3. Inflammatory causes

   Infectious causes, eg, tuberculosis, Whipple disease

   Chemical causes, eg, talc peritonitis

   Immunologic disorders, eg, systemic lupus erythematosus, vasculitis

   Allergic causes, eg, eosinophilic gastroenteritis

4. Miscellaneous causes

   Nephrotic syndrome

   Dialysis-associated ascites

   Ovarian hyperstimulation syndrome

   Thoracic duct obstruction

fluid.[15] An obese abdomen can masquerade as ascites, and an abdominal ultrasonogram may be required to establish the presence of ascites in an obese patient. An abdominal ultrasonogram is usually performed in patients with ascites not only to assess the presence of ascites and a mass, but also to investigate the hepatic echogenicity and vasculature.

Assessment of the Severity of Ascites

The International Ascites Club classifies ascites according to severity, complication, and response to diuretic treatment. Ascites can be classified into grade 1 (mild), grade 2 (moderate), and grade 3 (large) according to severity; into uncomplicated according to absence of complication; and into diuretic-resistant and diuretic-intractable according to the response to diuretic treatment (**Table 1**).[5,16,17]

Laboratory Studies Including Ascites Fluid Analysis

History and physical examination are important first steps in establishing the diagnosis of new-onset ascites, which should be further confirmed by an abdominal paracentesis and ultrasonography (**Box 2**). The presence of cirrhosis can be further assessed by measuring tests of liver function such as the serum bilirubin, albumin, and international normalized ratio (INR). These are often abnormal in patients with cirrhosis, although it is possible to have ascites as a result of cirrhosis in the presence of near normal values of these parameters. It is important to check renal function (serum creatinine) to establish a baseline and to determine if functional renal insufficiency is present. It is also worth remembering that a serum creatinine of 1.5 mg/dL, which is often considered to be near normal, represents considerable decrease in glomerular filtration in patients with cirrhosis who have decreased muscle mass. The presence of an underlying hepatocellular cancer should be sought with imaging studies and an alpha fetoprotein test. Endoscopy is sometimes performed to look for varices as further corroborative evidence for the presence of portal hypertension in cases where the diagnosis is not clear-cut. Similarly, a liver biopsy is performed in selected patients with ascites and liver disease of unknown etiology. Abdominal ultrasonography, CT, or MRI is used to image the liver to screen for hepatocellular carcinoma, portal vein thrombosis, and hepatic vein thrombosis.

Appropriate ascitic fluid analysis is probably the most efficient and effective method of diagnosing the cause of ascites.[15,18] The left lower quadrant of the abdomen, 2 finger breadths cephalad and 2 finger breadths medial to the anterior superior iliac crest, is the best location for paracentesis because it has thinner abdominal wall and larger pool of fluid accumulation.[19] The prothrombin time is often prolonged (approximately 71%) in patients with cirrhosis; however, the risk for bleeding is less than 1% after paracentesis in these patients even without any interventions to correct the coagulopathy.[20] The possibility for more serious complications such as hemoperitoneum and bowel perforation is remote, and they occur in less than 0.1% of patients.[21] Coagulopathy should preclude paracentesis only when there is clinical evidence of fibrinolysis or disseminated intravascular coagulation.[20]

In light of the presence of spontaneous bacterial peritonitis (SBP) in approximately 15% of hospitalized patients with cirrhosis and ascites, all such patients should be screened for SBP at the time of admission to the hospital.[22–25] Ascitic fluid should be analyzed in patients with new-onset ascites.[2] Ascitic fluid analysis to detect SBP is required in all patients with any evidence of clinical deterioration such as fever, abdominal pain, gastrointestinal bleeding, hepatic encephalopathy, hypotension, or renal failure.[26] The SAAG has been proven superior to the total-protein-based

Table 1
Classification of ascites according to severity, complication, and response to diuretic treatment

Severity			Uncomplicated	Refractory	
Grade 1 (Mild)	Grade 2 (Moderate)	Grade 3 (Large)		Diuretic-Resistant	Diuretic-Intractable
Ascites is only diagnosed on ultrasonography	Clinically sensiblemoderate distension of abdomen	Clinically marked or tense distension of abdomen	Ascites that is not complicated with infection and hepatorenal syndrome	Ascites is unresponsive to sodium restricted diet and high-dose diuretic treatment	Diuretic-induced adverse effects preclude the use of an effective diuretic dosage

---

Box 2
Evaluation of a patient with cirrhosis and ascites

General evaluation

    Complete blood count, platelets

Evaluation of liver disease

    Serum bilirubin, AST, ALT, alkaline phosphatase, serum albumin

    Prothrombin time, INR

    Tests to determine cause of liver disease, eg, hepatitis C antibody

    Upper abdominal imaging by ultrasonogram/CT scan[a]

    Esophagogastroduodenoscopy

    MELD score

Evaluation of renal functions

    Serum creatinine and electrolytes

    Urinalysis including microscopic examination

    24-h urinary sodium and/or protein[b]

Ascitic fluid analysis

    Cell count

    Bacterial culture with bedside inoculation into blood culture bottle

    Total protein and albumin

    Glucose, lactate dehydrogenase, amylase, triglycerides, and cytology, if indicated according to clinical situation[c]

[a] To look for hepatocellular cancer or portal vein thrombosis.
[b] Usually done if urinalysis indicates proteinurea or if noncompliance with sodium restriction is suspected.
[c] Usually glucose, albumin, and protein are the only routinely performed tests initially. The other tests are done if a diagnostic dilemma is present.

---

exudate/transudate analysis in categorizing ascites in prospective studies and has replaced the total-protein-based exudate/transudate concept in clinical practice.[14,27]

Calculation of SAAG is performed by measuring same-day albumin concentrations of serum and ascitic fluid and then subtracting the ascitic fluid albumin value from the serum albumin value. A SAAG value greater than or equal to 1.1 g/dL (11 g/L) predicts ascites as a result of portal hypertension with approximately 97% accuracy.[14] A SAAG greater than or equal to 1.1 g/dL may also be present in medical conditions such as congestive heart failure, Budd-Chiari syndrome, and portal hypertension—a second cause for ascites formation.[14,17] A SAAG less than 1.1 g/dL occurs commonly in peritoneal carcinomatosis, peritoneal tuberculosis, pancreatitis, serositis, and nephrotic syndrome.[14,17]

When there is no evidence of perforation of an intra-abdominal viscus or inflammation of intra-abdominal organs, an ascitic fluid neutrophil count greater than or equal to 250 cells/ mm^3 confirms the diagnosis of SBP.[15,16,28] The cell count is the most helpful parameter in diagnosing SBP. A urine dipstick is a quick test to detect neutrophil in ascites and may provide an early suspicion of SBP at bedside.[29,30] Gram stain of ascitic fluid is not necessary because it is rarely helpful.[31] When culture of ascitic fluid is performed, the fluid should be inoculated in blood culture bottles as opposed to sterile culture vials. In sterile vials, growth of an organism is noted in about 50% of cases whereas culture of ascitic fluid in blood culture bottles increases the probability of identification of an organism to about 80%.[32,33]

Cell count and differential, albumin, total protein concentration, and SAAG are tested in the initial screening of ascitic fluid if the ascites is believed to be likely uncomplicated on clinical grounds. Further testing is needed if the results of these tests are abnormal. Cell count and differential are usually adequate in patients receiving serial outpatient therapeutic paracentesis.[15] Lactate dehydrogenase, total protein, and glucose may help differentiate spontaneous from secondary bacterial peritonitis.[34] Ascitic fluid carcinoembryonic antigen (CEA) and alkaline phosphatase levels are useful for the differentiation of primary from secondary bacterial peritonitis with intestinal perforation. An ascitic fluid CEA greater than 5 ng/mL or ascitic fluid alkaline phosphatase values greater than 240 IU/L suggest gut perforation into ascitic fluid.[35] A high amylase level in ascitic fluid is diagnostic of pancreatic ascites. Ascitic fluid amylase should be determined whenever there is an increased clinical suspicion for pancreatic disease.[36–38] It is usually accompanied by increased total protein levels and decreased SAAG.

Bloody ascites with red blood cell count greater than 50,000 cells/mm^3 occurs in approximate 2% of patients with liver cirrhosis.[39] Hepatocellular carcinoma is the cause of bloody ascites in about 30% of patients with cirrhosis. However, the cause of bloody ascites cannot be found in about 50% of the cases. In patients with decompensated cirrhosis, cancer antigen 125 (CA 125) is usually elevated in both blood and ascites in proportion to the degree of ascites and does not necessarily indicate carcinoma as the underlying cause of ascites.[40–42]

Ascitic fluid cytology is an expensive test and has a low yield if it is not used in selective patients. One study showed that only 7% ascitic fluid cytologies are positive.[43] In peritoneal carcinomatosis, if adequate concentrated ascitic samples are sent and processed promptly, it is highly positive. The sensitivity of cytology in detecting peritoneal carcinomatosis is 96.7% if 3 samples are sent.[43] Breast, colon, gastric, or pancreatic carcinoma is usually the underlying cause of peritoneal carcinomatosis. Mycobacteria in ascitic fluid are difficult to detect. Smears for mycobacteria usually do not work, with sensitivity approaching 0%; however, the sensitivity of ascitic fluid culture for mycobacteria is approximately 50%.[44] Patients with high pretest probability for tuberculous peritonitis should be tested for mycobacteria on the first ascitic fluid sample.[45] Laparoscopy with peritoneal biopsy and mycobacterial culture of tubercles are the most rapid and accurate methods of diagnosing tuberculous peritonitis.

TREATMENT
General Management

The fundamental goal of ascites management is to induce a negative sodium balance (**Box 3**). Activation of sympathetic nervous system, RAAS, and ADH play an important role in the pathophysiology of ascites formation. Physiologically, an upright position activates these systems that theoretically worsen sodium and fluid retention and decrease response to diuretics in patients with cirrhosis and ascites.[46,47] Moderate physical activity may induce more profound effects on these systems.[48,49] These findings support the traditional practice to recommend bed rest as part of the treatment for ascites. However, bed rest is impractical, especially in patients with mild and moderate ascites. Another concern is that bed rest may further decondition the patient, weaken physical strength, and induce muscle atrophy in patients with

---

Box 3
Treatment of ascites

1. General measures:

   a. Sodium restriction

   b. Maintain caloric intake at goal

   c. Protein intake (1 g/kg/d unless patient is severely encephalopathic or catabolic)

   d. Immunization: pneumococcal vaccine, influenza vaccine

2. Treatment of underlying liver disease:

   a. Alcohol abstinence

   b. Hepatitis B: antiviral therapy for E antigen positive subjects

   c. Hemochromatosis: phlebotomy

   d. Wilson disease: chelation therapy

3. Standard medical treatment (diuretics + paracentesis):

   a. Distal tubule acting diuretics, eg, spironolactone

   b. Loop-acting diuretics, eg, furosemide

   c. Large volume paracentesis (>5 L)

4. Transjugular intrahepatic portasystemic shunts (TIPS)

5. Peritoneovenous shunts

6. Liver transplantation

---

cirrhosis and ascites. There are no controlled trials to support the theory of bed rest. Therefore, bed rest is not generally recommended for the management of patients with uncomplicated ascites.[17]

Dietary sodium restriction and oral diuretics are mainstays of treatment for patients with cirrhosis and ascites. Stringent dietary sodium restriction mobilizes ascites in patients with portal hypertension. Negative sodium balance leads to fluid and weight loss in patients with cirrhosis and ascites. It is usually sodium restriction, not water restriction, that induces weight loss, because water follows sodium passively.[50] Dietary sodium should be restricted to 2000 mg/d (88 mmol/d). Nonurinary excretion of sodium is about 10 mmol/d. One of the goals of treatment is to achieve negative sodium balance. In order to achieve negative sodium balance, urinary sodium excretion should be greater than 78 mmol/d. If weight loss is not as expected, measurement of urinary sodium excretion may be helpful.[18] Collection of 24-hour urine for sodium measurement is cumbersome. Random urine "spot" sodium concentration is a more quick and convenient method to determine urinary excretion with 97% accuracy.[51] Sodium restriction is effective in reducing the dose of diuretics, providing faster solution for ascites, and a shorter hospital stay.[52,53] However, dietary sodium restriction is successful in achieving a negative sodium balance in only about 10% to 15% of patients with cirrhosis and ascites.[54] Compliance with sodium restriction is a practical issue in daily management of patients with cirrhosis and ascites because most patients are reluctant to go along with sodium restriction alone. There are no controlled trials regarding fluid restriction. Most experts believe fluid restriction has no role in the management of patients with uncomplicated ascites.[15,17] Water restriction is recommended only when the serum sodium decreases to values below 130 mEq/L.

Consideration should be given to treatment of the underlying cause of cirrhosis, particularly for alcohol-related and hepatitis B–related cirrhosis. Abstinence can result in dramatic improvement in liver function and even resolve ascites in the course of a few months in patients with alcoholic hepatitis and cirrhosis. The benefits of abstinence are seen in patients with alcoholic liver disease and cirrhosis of varying severity.[55,56]

A nutritionist can play an important role in providing education regarding salt and caloric intake. Protein-calorie malnutrition and weight loss are common among patients with cirrhosis and ascites. Such patients often complain of dyspeptic symptoms such as early satiety, nausea, and postprandial fullness. A study has reported significant reduction in median postprandial gastric volume and gastric accommodation; and paracentesis improves fasting gastric volume, tolerance to ingestion of maximum volume, and caloric intake.[57] Decreased oral intake and absorption of nutrients, increased energy expenditure, and altered fuel metabolism with a starvation pattern of metabolism are the underlying mechanisms for malnutrition in patients with cirrhosis and ascites.[58–60] Nutritional therapy with improved nutritional status may reduce the occurrence of infection and perioperative morbidity. Although there are no studies that show the value of nutritional status correction to improve ascites management and hard outcomes such as mortality, absence of evidence does not indicate the absence of an effect. One can imagine that good nutritional support may be essential to make the patient a good candidate for liver transplant. Supplemental enteral nutrition is needed in patients with severe malnutrition and may improve liver function and hepatic encephalopathy.[58–61]

Specific therapies for ascites

Diuretics have been the mainstay of treatment for patients with cirrhosis and ascites since they first became available. Patients with grade 1 ascites have mild ascites that can only be detected by ultrasound. These patients should have a sodium-restricted diet but do not require diuretics. Patients with grade 2 or higher severity require diuretics to reduce edema and ascites. Activation of RAAS plays an important role in the development of ascites. Spironolactone is the diuretic of choice because it is an aldosterone antagonist that acts on the distal tubules in the kidney to increase sodium excretion and conserve potassium. As a single agent, spironolactone has been shown to be more efficacious than furosemide in a randomized clinical trial.[62] However, it is used as a single agent mostly in patients with minimal fluid overload.[63]

Furosemide is a loop diuretic that causes marked natruresis and diuresis. It is less efficacious than spironolactone as a single agent in the treatment of patients with cirrhosis and ascites.[62] It is usually used as an adjunct to spironolactone treatment. It should be used with caution because it can cause hyponatremia, hypokalemia, and prerenal renal failure. Because of its good oral availability and intravenous administration–induced acute reduction in renal glomerular filtration rate, furosemide is usually used as an oral agent.[64,65] Simultaneous use of spironolactone and furosemide increases the natriuretic effect and prevents hypokalemia.[15] Furosemide 40 mg and spironolactone 100 mg daily are usually started as an initial dose in patients with moderate to severe ascites. It usually takes 3 to 5 days for the diuretics to show their maximal effects.[66] The doses of spironolactone and furosemide can be increased simultaneously in a stepwise manner until the maximal doses of 400 mg spironolactone and 160 mg furosemide every day are reached if desired weight loss and natriuresis are not attained.[15,18]

Dietary sodium restriction should always be implemented together with the use of diuretics. The desired rate of daily weight loss depends upon the severity of edema.

In patients with severe edema, diuretics can be given to patients with cirrhosis and ascites without limitation of daily weight loss. Once ascites has resolved, daily maximal weight loss of 0.5 kg is probably a reasonable goal.[67] This approach of dual diuretics regimen in combination with dietary sodium restriction has been used successfully in achieving improvement of ascites to an acceptable level in more than 90% of patients in a large, multicenter, randomized, controlled clinical trial.[68] Efforts should be made to avoid overdiuresis that can lead to decreased intravascular volume, prerenal kidney impairment, hepatic encephalopathy, and hyponatremia.[69] Serum creatinine greater than 2.0 mg/dL, or serum sodium less than 120 mmol/L indicate that diuretics should be discontinued and alternative treatment considered.[15] The hepatic encephalopathy associated with volume contraction is best treated with albumin infusions. In patients with cirrhosis who have ascites, side effects of spironolactone include hyperkalemia and decreased libido, impotence, and gynecomastia in men and menstrual irregularity in women, as a result of its antiandrogenic activity. Patients with organic renal disease may not tolerate spironolactone because of hyperkalemia, a serious complication that frequently limits its use in such a situation. Amiloride may be considered as an alternative in patients with tender gynecomastia, but it was shown to be more expensive and less effective than spironolactone in a randomized controlled clinical study.[65] Tamoxifen at a dose of 20 mg twice daily has been reported to be effective in managing the gynecomastia.[63]

Clonidine is a centrally acting alpha-2 agonist that has sympatholytic activity in patients with cirrhosis.[70–72] Simultaneous administration of clonidine and spironolactone has been shown in studies to increase natriuresis and body weight loss more efficiently, to induce an earlier diuretic response, and fewer complications such as hyperkalemia and renal impairment.[73–75] Diuretic use is one of the underlying causes of muscle cramps. In patients with cirrhosis and ascites receiving diuretic therapy, muscle cramps may require a reduction in diuretic dosage. Quinidine sulfate at a dose of 400 mg daily or intravenous albumin at 25 g/wk reduces the frequency and severity of diuretic-induced muscle cramps in patients with cirrhosis and ascites.[76,77]

Therapeutic paracentesis

Diuretics alone may be inadequate in managing patients with large or refractory ascites. Therapeutic paracentesis does not correct the underlying pathophysiological process that results in ascites formation in patients with cirrhosis but usually relieves symptoms caused by abdominal tension. In prospective studies the safety of a single 5 L or less paracentesis without postprocedure colloid infusion for intravascular volume expansion has been shown.[78,79] Large volume paracentesis (LVP) can be performed safely with the administration of intravenous albumin infusion (8 g/L of ascites removed).[80] LVP with intravenous albumin infusion rapidly removed ascites, was more effective in maintaining an ascites-free state, and was associated with fewer complications and shorter hospital stay when compared with diuretic therapy.[69,81] Total paracentesis followed by postparacentesis volume expansion with albumin is as safe as serial LVP alone.[78,80]

A complication of LVP is the development of postparacentesis circulatory dysfunction.[82] This is characterized by worsening vasodilation, hyponatremia, activation of sodium-retentive hormones and sometimes azotemia. It is a marker for poorer outcomes and can be partially prevented by the use of albumin given intravenously at a dose of 6 to 8 g per liter of ascites removed.[83] Although albumin was formerly thought to be a simple volume expander, it is now thought that albumin may have important effects on the endothelial dysfunction and circulatory disturbances associated with cirrhosis.[84]

Transjugular intrahepatic portosystemic shunts
These procedures decompress the portal vein by providing a low-resistance channel between the intrahepatic portion of the portal vein and the hepatic vein. They increase venous return to the heart and improve the effective circulating volume. This leads to improved renal perfusion and a decrease in renal tubular sodium reabsorption, thereby causing a natriuresis. Transjugular intrahepatic portosystemic shunts (TIPS) effectively removes ascites and maintains an ascites-free state. However, these benefits are offset by an increased incidence of hepatic encephalopathy.[85,86] The incidence of hospitalization and overall survival are not impacted by TIPS. The outcomes after TIPS depend on the model end-stage liver disease (MELD) score.[87] The ideal candidate for TIPS is one who has relatively preserved hepatic synthetic function and renal function and who is free of encephalopathy.

Peritoneovenous shunts
A peritoneovenous shunt has been used for the treatment of refractory ascites. It also increases the central volume and induces diuresis. Although as effective as repeated LVP, it does not improve survival. Enthusiasm for this procedure has waned because of the increased risk of complications, such as disseminated intravascular coagulation, infection, and occlusion of the subclavian vein and superior vena cava, which can preclude a liver transplant.

Management of uncomplicated ascites
This is usually managed with a combination of general measures and the use of diuretics and sodium restriction. Initially when patients present with moderate or severe ascites, a LVP is done to make the patients comfortable and then sodium restriction and diuretics are used to maintain an ascites-free state. Although this is effective in most patients, some patients progress to the refractory ascites state. Only liver transplant provides long-term survival in patients with end-stage liver disease, and in the absence of an obvious contraindication to transplantation, such patients should be referred expeditiously to a transplant center.

Management of refractory ascites
Diuretic refractory ascites (see **Table 1**), that is, ascites that does not respond to maximal diuretic doses, is associated with increasing systemic vasodilation and activation of systemic sodium and water retentive mechanisms. Increasing vasodilation decreases effective circulating volume and renal perfusion. This decreases delivery of the drugs to their site of action (the distal tubule for spironolactone and the lumen of the loop of Henle for furosemide) and causes diuretic resistance.

Repeated LVP or TIP are the most commonly used modalities for the treatment of refractory ascites. Although they relieve ascites immediately, they are associated with recurrence of ascites in most patients and do not improve survival. Repeated LVP is associated with discomfort, protein loss and malnutrition, the need for repeated hospitalization, and health care resource utilization. It is, however, a relatively inexpensive approach.

TIPS is substantially superior to LVP for long-term control of ascites (**Fig. 2**).[86] This does not translate to improved survival and the decrease in ascites-related health care resource utilization is offset by increased encephalopathy-related morbidity. Also, for the same survival outcomes, TIPS is less cost-effective than LVP. Hyperbilirubinemia, severe hypoprothrombinemia, and renal failure are risk factors associated with a poor

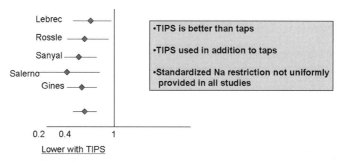

Fig. 2. A meta-analysis of TIPS versus LVP shows TIPS to be superior to LVP for control of ascites as shown by the odds ratio in individual studies. (*Data from* Albillos A, Bañares R, González M, et al. A meta-analysis of transjugular intrahepatic portosystemic shunt versus paracentesis for refractory ascites. J Hepatol 2005;43:990–6.)

outcome after TIPS.[87] Although TIPS is better than LVP for control of ascites in general,[88] the outcomes of TIPS for refractory ascites are best in those who have failed repeated LVP and who have relatively preserved liver and renal function (ie, a creatinine less than 1.5 mg/dL, INR less than 1.5, and bilirubin less than 2 mg/dL). Ideally, it should be used as a bridge to liver transplant.

Hyponatremia is another major management challenge in patients with cirrhosis and ascites. It occurs in about 50% of patients with cirrhosis and is associated with increased mortality (**Fig. 3**).[89] It is generally managed by volume restriction. There are anecdotal reports of improvement with albumin infusions as well. The role of aquaretic drugs in the management of ascites-related hyponatremia is under investigation.

Spontaneous bacterial peritonitis
SBP should always be considered in the differential diagnosis when a patient with cirrhosis and ascites develops fever, abdominal pain, altered mental status, variceal hemorrhage, or azotemia. It is diagnosed by a diagnostic paracentesis and treated with a third-generation cephalosporin.[90] A 5-day course has been found to be as effective as a 10-day course for uncomplicated SBP.[91] Typically, treatment is switched to oral quinolone therapy after 3 to 5 days of intravenous antibiotics. SBP recurs frequently and secondary prophylaxis with oral quinolones is effective in

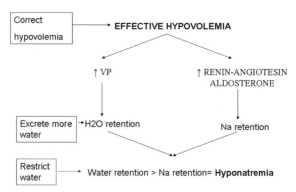

Fig. 3. A pathophysiology-based approach to the treatment of hyponatremia associated with cirrhosis.

preventing recurrence and is therefore recommended.[92] Primary prophylaxis for SBP should be considered in those with low-protein ascites and severe hepatic synthetic dysfunction.[93]

REFERENCES

1. Hernandez-Guerra M, Garcia-Pagan JC, Bosch J. Increased hepatic resistance: a new target in the pharmacologic therapy of portal hypertension. J Clin Gastroenterol 2005;39:131–7.
2. Gines P, Cardenas A, Arroyo V, et al. Management of cirrhosis and ascites. N Engl J Med 2004;350:1646–54.
3. Moller S, Bendtsen F, Henriksen JH. Pathophysiological basis of pharmacotherapy in the hepatorenal syndrome. Scand J Gastroenterol 2005;40:491–500.
4. Schrier RW, Arroyo V, Bernardi M, et al. Peripheral arterial vasodilation hypothesis: a proposal for the initiation of renal sodium and water retention in cirrhosis. Hepatology 1988;8:1151–7.
5. Arroyo V, Ginès P, Gerbes AL, et al. Definition and diagnostic criteria of refractory ascites and hepatorenal syndrome in cirrhosis. Hepatology 1996;23:164–76.
6. Oben JA, Diehl AM. Sympathetic nervous system regulation of liver repair. Anat Rec A Discov Mol Cell Evol Biol 2004;280:874–83.
7. Arroyo V, Gines P. Mechanism of sodium retention and ascites formation in cirrhosis. J Hepatol 1993;17:24–8.
8. Jimenez-Saenz M, Soria IC, Bernardez JR, et al. Renal sodium retention in portal hypertension and hepatorenal reflex: from practice to science. Hepatology 2003;37:1494–5.
9. Iwakiri Y, Groszmann R. The hyperdynamic circulation of chronic liver diseases: from the patient to the molecule. Hepatology 2006;43:S121–31.
10. Iwakiri Y, Groszmann R. Vascular endothelial dysfunction in cirrhosis. J Hepatol 2007;46:927–34.
11. Wiest R, Das S, Cadelina G. Bacterial translocation in cirrhotic rats stimulates eNOS-derived NO production and impairs mesenteric vascular contractility. J Clin Invest 1999;104:1223–33.
12. Wiest R, Garcia-Tsao G. Bacterial translocation (BT) in cirrhosis. Hepatology 2005;41:422–33.
13. Riordan SM, Williams R. The intestinal flora and bacterial infection in cirrhosis. J Hepatol 2006;45:744–57.
14. Runyon BA, Montano AA, Akriviadis EA, et al. The serum-ascites albumin gradient is superior to the exudate-transudate concept in the differential diagnosis of ascites. Ann Intern Med 1992;117:215–20.
15. Runyon BA. Management of adult patients with ascites due to cirrhosis. Hepatology 2004;39:1–16.
16. Moore KP, Wong F, Ginès P. The management of ascites in cirrhosis: report on the consensus conference of the International Ascites Club. Hepatology 2003;38:258–66.
17. Moore KP, Aithal GP. Guidelines on the management of ascites in cirrhosis. Gut 2006;55(Suppl 6):vi1–12.
18. Runyon BA. Care of patient with ascites. N Engl J Med 1994;330:337–42.
19. Sakai H, Mendler MH, Runyon BA. The left lower quadrant is the best site for paracentesis: an ultrasound evaluation. Hepatology 2002;36:525A [abstract].
20. Runyon BA. Paracentesis of ascetic fluid: a safe procedure. Arch Intern Med 1986;146:2259–61.

21. Webster ST, Brown KL, Lucey MR, et al. Hemorrhagic complications of large volume abdominal paracentesis. Am J Gastroenterol 1996;92:366–8.
22. Caly WR, Strauss E. A prospective study of bacterial infections in patients with cirrhosis. J Hepatol 1993;18:353–8.
23. Bac D-J, Siersema PD, Mulder PGH, et al. Spontaneous bacterial peritonitis: outcome and predictive factors. Eur J Gastroenterol Hepatol 1993;5:635–40.
24. Rimola A, Garcia-Tsao G, Navasa M, et al. Diagnosis, treatment and prophylaxis of spontaneous bacterial peritonitis: a consensus document. J Hepatol 2000;32: 142–53.
25. Pinzello G, Simonetti RG, Craxi A, et al. Spontaneous bacterial peritonitis: a prospective investigation in predominantly nonalcoholic patients. Hepatology 1983;3:545–9.
26. Ginès P, Cárdenas A. The management of ascites and hyponatremia in cirrhosis. Semin Liver Dis 2008;28:43–58.
27. Hooefs JC. Serum protein concentration and portal pressure determine the ascitic fluid protein concentration in patients with chronic liver disease. J Lab Clin Med 1983;102:260–73.
28. Ghassemi S, Garcia-Tsao G. Prevention and treatment of infections in patients with cirrhosis. Best Pract Res Clin Gastroenterol 2007;21:77–93.
29. Castellote J, Lopez C, Gornals J, et al. Rapid diagnosis of spontaneous bacterial peritonitis by use of reagent strip. Hepatology 2003;37:893–6.
30. Runyon BA. Strips and tubes: refining the diagnosis of spontaneous bacterial peritonitis. Hepatology 2003;37:745–7.
31. Runyon BA, Canwati HN, Akriviadis EA. Optimization of ascetic fluid culture technique. Gastroenterology 1988;95:1351–5.
32. Runyon BA, Antillon MR, Akriviadis EA, et al. Bedside inoculation of blood culture bottles is superior to delayed inoculation in the detection of spontaneous bacterial peritonitis. J Clin Microbiol 1990;28:2811–2.
33. Castellote J, Xiol X, Verdaguer R, et al. Comparison of two ascetic fluid culture methods in cirrhotic patients with spontaneous bacterial peritonitis. Am J Gastroenterol 1990;85:1605–8.
34. Akriviadis EA, Runyon BA. The value of an algorithm in differentiating spontaneous from secondary bacterial peritonitis. Gastroenterology 1990;98: 127–33.
35. Wu SS, Lin OS, Chen Y-Y, et al. Ascitic fluid carcinoembryonic antigen and alkaline phosphatase levels for the differentiation of primary from secondary bacterial peritonitis with intestinal perforation. J Hepatol 2001;34:215–21.
36. Runyon BA. Amylase levels in ascetic fluid. J Clin Gastroenterol 1987;9:172–4.
37. Polak M, Mattosinho Francis LC. Chronic pancreatitis with massive ascites. Digestion 1968;1:296–304.
38. Schindler SC, Schaefer JW, Hull D, et al. Chronic pancreatic ascites. Gastroenterology 1970;59:453–9.
39. DeSitter L, Rector WG Jr. The significance of bloody ascites in patients with cirrhosis. Am J Gastroenterol 1984;95:1351–5.
40. Molina R, Filella X, Bruix J, et al. Cancer antigen 125 in serum and ascitic fluid of patients with liver diseases. Clin Chem 1991;37:1379–83.
41. Zuckerman E, Lanir A, Sabo E, et al. Cancer antigen 125: a sensitive marker of ascites in patients with liver cirrhosis. Am J Gastroenterol 1999;94:1613–8.
42. Sari R, Yildirim B, Sevinc A, et al. Sensitity of cancer antigen 125 in patients with liver cirrhosis in the presence of ascites [Erratum in Am J Gastroenterol 2001; 96: 1319]. Am J Gastroenterol 2001;96:253–4.

43. Runyon BA, Hoefs JC, Morgan TR. Ascitic fluid analysis in malignancy-related ascites. Hepatology 1988;8:1104–9.
44. Hillebrand DJ, Runyon BA, Yasmineh WG, et al. Ascitic fluid adenosine deaminase insensitivity in detecting tuberculous peritonitis in the United States. Hepatology 1996;24(140):1408–12.
45. Cappell MS, Shetty V. A multicenter, case-controlled study of the clinical presentation and etiology of ascites and of the safety and efficacy of diagnostic abdominal paracentesis in HIV seropositive patients. Am J Gastroenterol 1994;89:2172–7.
46. Gines P, Fernandez-Esparrach G, Arroyo V, et al. Pathogenesis of ascites in cirrhosis. Semin Liver Dis 1997;17:175–89.
47. Ring-Larsen H, Henriksen JH, Wilken C, et al. Diuretic treatment in decompensated cirrhosis and congestive heart failure: effect of posture. BMJ 1986;292:1351–3.
48. Salo J, Gines A, Anibarro L, et al. Effect of upright posture and physical exercise on endogenous neurohumoral systems in cirrhotic patients with sodium retention and normal supine plasma renin, aldosterone, and norepinephrine levels. Hepatology 1995;22:479–87.
49. Salo J, Guevara M, Fernandez-Esparrach G, et al. Impairment of renal function during moderate physical exercise in cirrhotic patients with ascites: relationship with the activity of neurohormonal systems. Hepatology 1997;25:1338–42.
50. Eisenmenger WJ, Ahrens EH, Blondheim SH, et al. The effect of rigid sodium restriction in patients with cirrhosis of the liver and ascites. J Lab Clin Med 1949;34:1029–38.
51. Stiehm AJ, Mendler MH, Runyon BA. Detection of diuretic-resistance or diuretic-sensitivity by the spot urine Na/K ratio in 729 specimens from cirrhotics with ascites: approximately 90% accuracy as compared to 24-hr urine Na excretion. Hepatology 2002;36:222A [abstract].
52. Descos L, Gauthier A, Levy VG, et al. Comparison of six treatments of ascites in patients with liver cirrhosis. Hepatogastroenterology 1983;30:15–20.
53. Gauthier A, Levy VG, Quinton A, et al. Salt or no salt in the treatment of cirrhotic ascites: a randomised study. Gut 1986;27:705–9.
54. Gerbes AL. Medical treatment of ascites in cirrhosis. J Hepatol 1993;17:S4–9.
55. Runyon BA. Ascites and spontaneous bacterial peritonitis. In: Feldman M, Friedman LS, Sleisenger MH, editors. Sleisenger and Fordtran's gastrointestinal and liver disease. 7th edition. Philadelphia: Saunders; 2002. p. 1517–42.
56. Veldt BJ, Laine F, Guillogomarc'h A, et al. Indication of liver transplantation in severe alcoholic liver cirrhosis: quantitative evaluation and optimal timing. J Hepatol 2002;36:93–8.
57. Aqel BA, Scolapio JS, Dickson RC, et al. Contribution of ascites to impaired gastric function and nutritional intake in patients with cirrhosis and ascites. Clin Gastroenterol Hepatol 2005;3:1095–100.
58. Henkel AS, Buchman AL. Nutritional support in patients with chronic liver disease. Nat Clin Pract Gastroenterol Hepatol 2006;3:202–9.
59. McCullough AJ. Nutrition and malnutrition in liver disease. In: Wolfe MM, Davis GL, Farraye F, et al, editors. Therapy of digestive disorders. 2nd edition. Philadelphia: Saunders; 2006. p. 67–83.
60. Kearns PJ, Young H, Garcia G. Accelerated improvement of alcoholic liver disease with enteral nutrition. Gastroenterology 1992;102:200–5.
61. Cabrè E, Gonzalez-Hux F, Abad-Lacruz A. Effect of total enteral nutrition on the short-term outcome of severely malnourished cirrhotics: a randomized controlled trial. Gastroenterology 1990;98:715–20.

62. Perez-Ayuso RM, Arroyo V, Planas R, et al. Randomized comparative study of efficacy of furosemide vs. spironolactone in nonazotemic cirrhosis with ascites. Gastroenterology 1983;84:961–8.

63. Sungaila I, Bartle WR, Walker SE, et al. Spironolactone pharmacokinetics and pharmacodynamics in patients with cirrhotic ascites. Gastroenterology 1992; 102:1680–5.

64. Daskalopoulos G, Laffi G, Morgan T, et al. Immediate effects of furosemide on renal hemodynamics in chronic liver disease with ascites. Gastroenterology 1987;92:1859–63.

65. Angeli P, Pria MD, De Bei E, et al. Randomized clinical study of the efficacy of amiloride and potassium canrenoate in nonazotemic cirrhotic patients with ascites. Hepatology 1994;19:72–9.

66. Karim A. Spironolactone metabolism in man revisited. In: Brunner HR, editor. Contemporary trends in diuretic therapy. Amsterdam: Excerpta Medica; 1986. p. 22–37.

67. Pockros PJ, Reynolds TB. Rapid diuresis in patients with ascites from chronic liver disease: the importance of peripheral edema. Gastroenterology 1986;90: 1827–33.

68. Stanley MM, Ochi S, Lee KK, et al. Peritoneovenous shunting as compared with medical treatment in patients with alcoholic cirrhosis and massive ascites. N Engl J Med 1989;321:1632–8.

69. Gines P, Arroyo V, Quintero E, et al. Comparison of paracentesis and diuretics in the treatment of cirrhotics with tense ascites: results of a randomized study. Gastroenterology 1987;93:234–41.

70. Moreau R, Lec SS, Hadengue A, et al. Hemodynamic effects of a clonidine-induced decrease in sympathetic tone in patients with cirrhosis. Hepatology 1987;7:149–54.

71. Esler M, Dudley F, Jennings G, et al. Increased sympathetic nervous activity and the effects of its inhibition with clonidine in alcoholic cirrhosis. Ann Intern Med 1992;116:446–55.

72. Roulot D, Moreau R, Gaudin C, et al. Long term sympathetic and hemodynamic responses to clonidine in patients with cirrhosis. Gastroenterology 1992;102: 1309–18.

73. Lenaerts A, Van Cauter J, Moukhaiber H, et al. Treatment of refractory ascites with clonidine and spironolactone. Gastroenterol Clin Biol 1997;21:524–5.

74. Lenaerts A, Codden T, Van Cauter J, et al. Interest of the association clonidine-spironolactone in cirrhotic patients with ascites and activation of sympathetic nervous system. Acta Gastroenterol Belg 2002;65:1–5.

75. Lenaerts A, Codden T, Meunier JD, et al. Effects of clonidine on diuretic response in ascitic patients with cirrhosis and activation of sympathetic nervous system. Hepatology 2006;44:844–9.

76. Lee FY, Lee SD, Hwang SJ, et al. A randomized controlled trial of quinidine in the treatment of cirrhotic patients with muscle cramps. J Hepatol 1991;12:236–40.

77. Angeli P, Albino G, Carraro P, et al. Cirrhosis and muscle cramps: evidence of a causal relationship. Hepatology 1996;23:264–73.

78. Peltekian KM, Wong F, Liu PP, et al. Cardiovascular, renal and neurohumoral responses to single large-volume paracentesis in cirrhotic patients with diuretic-resistant ascites. Am J Gastroenterol 1997;92:394–9.

79. Runyon BA. Patient selection is important in studying the impact of large-volume paracentesis on intravascular volume. Am J Gastroenterol 1997;92:371–3.

80. Tito L, Gines P, Arroyo V, et al. Total paracentesis associated with intravenous albumin management of patients with cirrhosis and ascites. Gastroenterology 1990;98:146–51.
81. Quintero E, Gines P, Arroyo V, et al. Paracentesis versus diuretics in the treatment of cirrhotics with tense ascites. Lancet 1985;16:611–2.
82. Ruiz-Del-Arbol L, Monescillo A, Jimenez W, et al. Paracentesis-induced circulatory dysfunction: mechanism and effect on hepatic hemodynamics in cirrhosis. Gastroenterology 1997;113:579–86.
83. Gines P, Tito L, Arroyo V, et al. Randomized comparative study of therapeutic paracentesis with and without intravenous albumin in cirrhosis. Gastroenterology 1988;94:1493–502.
84. Gines A, Fernandez-Esparrach G, Monescillo A, et al. Randomized trial comparing albumin, dextran 70, and polygeline in cirrhotic patients with ascites treated by paracentesis. Gastroenterology 1996;111:1002–10.
85. Wong F, Sniderman K, Liu P, et al. The mechanism of the initial natriuresis after transjugular intrahepatic portosystemic shunt. Gastroenterology 1997;112:899–907.
86. Sanyal AJ, Genning C, Reddy KR, et al. The North American Study for the Treatment of Refractory Ascites. Gastroenterology 2003;124:634–41.
87. Malinchoc M, Kamath PS, Gordon FD, et al. A model to predict poor survival in patients undergoing transjugular intrahepatic portosystemic shunts. Hepatology 2000;31:864–71.
88. Albillos A, Banares R, Gonzalez M, et al. A meta-analysis of transjugular intrahepatic portosystemic shunt versus paracentesis for refractory ascites. J Hepatol 2005;43:990–6.
89. Londono MC, Guevara M, Rimola A, et al. Hyponatremia impairs early posttransplantation outcome in patients with cirrhosis undergoing liver transplantation. Gastroenterology 2006;130:1135–43.
90. Garcia-Tsao G. Bacterial infections in cirrhosis. Can J Gastroenterol 2004;18:405–6.
91. Runyon BA, McHutchison JG, Antillon MR, et al. Short-course versus long-course antibiotic treatment of spontaneous bacterial peritonitis. A randomized controlled study of 100 patients. Gastroenterology 1991;100:1737–42.
92. Tito L, Rimola A, Gines P, et al. Recurrence of spontaneous bacterial peritonitis in cirrhosis: frequency and predictive factors. Hepatology 1988;8:27–31.
93. Fernandez J, Navasa M, Planas R, et al. Primary prophylaxis of spontaneous bacterial peritonitis delays hepatorenal syndrome and improves survival in cirrhosis. Gastroenterology 2007;133:818–24.

Hepatic Encephalopathy: Pathophysiology and Emerging Therapies

Vinay Sundaram, MD, Obaid S. Shaikh, MD, FRCP*

KEYWORDS

- Coma • Liver failure • Cirrhosis • Ammonia
- Neuropsychiatric dysfunction

Hepatic encephalopathy (HE) refers to neuropsychiatric abnormalities that result from hepatic dysfunction. It is one of the principal manifestations of chronic liver disease and a cardinal feature of fulminant hepatic failure. In patients with either acute or chronic liver disease, the presence and severity of HE are major determinants of prognosis. In a consensus statement, the working party at the 11th World Congresses of Gastroenterology (WCOG) proposed classification of HE into 3 types based on the nature of hepatic dysfunction with further categorization according to the pattern and severity of neurologic abnormalities.[1] Type A encephalopathy is associated with acute liver failure (ALF), type B with portosystemic bypass without intrinsic liver disease, and type C with cirrhosis. HE is subcategorized as episodic, persistent, or minimal. Episodic HE could be with or without precipitating factors (precipitated vs spontaneous) and recurrent if 2 or more episodes occur within a year. Persistent HE impairs social and occupational functioning and is subdivided into mild, severe, or treatment-dependent. Minimal encephalopathy is associated with cognitive dysfunction that is without overt symptoms. This review focuses on HE associated with cirrhosis (type C).

PATHOPHYSIOLOGY

The pathogenesis of HE in cirrhosis is complex and has multiple components, including ammonia, inflammatory cytokines, benzodiazepine-like compounds, and manganese, that cause functional impairment of neuronal cells.[2] Numerous factors have been shown to precipitate HE including infections, sedatives, gastrointestinal bleeding, dietary protein excess, diuretics, and electrolyte imbalance.[3]

Division of Gastroenterology, Hepatology and Nutrition, University of Pittsburgh School of Medicine, Pittsburgh, PA 15213, USA
* Corresponding author. Center for Liver Diseases, University of Pittsburgh Medical Center, Kaufmann Building, Suite 916, 3471 Fifth Avenue, Pittsburgh, PA 15213.
E-mail address: obaid@pitt.edu (O.S. Shaikh).

Med Clin N Am 93 (2009) 819–836
doi:10.1016/j.mcna.2009.03.009
0025-7125/09/$ – see front matter © 2009 Elsevier Inc. All rights reserved.

medical.theclinics.com

Ammonia

Ammonia is created primarily from nitrogenous products in the diet, bacterial metabolism of urea and proteins in the colon, and from deamination of glutamine in the small intestine by the enzyme glutaminase.[4] Ammonia is also produced by skeletal muscles, but how this contributes to HE has not been established. From the gut, ammonia enters the portal circulation and is converted to urea by the liver; the urea is subsequently excreted by the kidneys.[5]

Due to hepatocellular dysfunction and portosystemic collaterals in cirrhosis, the ammonia concentration rises in the bloodstream and crosses the blood-brain barrier (BBB). Exposure to ammonia results in structural alterations in neurons manifested primarily as astrocyte swelling.[3] Autopsy studies of brain tissue in cirrhotic patients have demonstrated swollen astrocytes with enlarged nuclei and displacement of chromatin to the perimeter of the cell, a condition known as Alzheimer type II astrocytosis.[6,7] One mechanism of neuronal edema has been attributed to accumulation of glutamine, known as the "Trojan horse" hypothesis.[8] Once ammonia enters the astrocytes, the enzyme glutamine synthetase facilitates its interaction with the excitatory neurotransmitter glutamate to form glutamine.[9] Glutamine enters the mitochondria and is subsequently cleaved by glutaminase to ammonia and glutamate, thereby increasing intracellular ammonia levels.[8] This causes a feed-forward loop as elevation in mitochondrial ammonia causes production of reactive nitrogen and oxygen species (RNOS) leading to further edema.[8,10–14] Studies have also examined the role of ammonia-induced potentiation of aquaporin-4, a water channel expressed copiously in astrocytes.[15] Astrocyte edema also causes depletion of taurine, a molecule that serves as an antioxidant and helps to buffer ammonia-induced toxicity.[16]

Increased ammonia levels cause abnormal cerebral blood flow and glucose metabolism. Single photon emission computed tomographic (SPECT) studies have demonstrated altered cerebral perfusion with hyperammonemia resulting in a redistribution of blood flow from the cortex to the subcortical regions, which was associated with impaired performance on neuropsychiatric testing.[17,18] Additional PET studies using ammonia as a tracer showed redistribution of glucose utilization within the brain.[19]

γ-Aminobutyric Acid Agonists

γ-Aminobutyric acid (GABA) acts as an inhibitory neurotransmitter. Increased "GABAergic tone" has been implicated in the pathogenesis of HE. The reasoning behind this notion initially came from reports of the beneficial effect of the benzodiazepine antagonist flumazenil.[20,21] There is an excess of benzodiazepine-like compounds in HE that are derived from synthesis by intestinal flora, vegetables in the diet, and medications.[22–24] Natural benzodiazepines may also accumulate in the brain.[25] Furthermore, the cirrhotic patient has poor ability to clear benzodiazepine-like compounds. Such compounds bind to the GABA receptor complex inducing GABA release and neuroinhibition. Ammonia itself may also bind to the GABA receptor complex.[26] In addition, it may potentiate benzodiazepines by upregulating expression of peripheral-type benzodiazepine receptors (PTBRs) that trigger synthesis of neurosteroids, which are strong GABA agonists.[27,28] Although studies have reported increased densities of benzodiazepine receptors in animal models of ALF,[29,30] the GABA receptor complex seems to be unchanged in cirrhotic patients.[31–33] Therefore, in patients with cirrhosis, GABAergic tone is more likely attributed to elevated levels of benzodiazepine-like compounds.

Inflammation

The development of HE is partially attributed to inflammation in view of the high prevalence of infections among patients with HE, the link between markers of systemic inflammatory response syndrome (SIRS) and HE, and the association of SIRS with deterioration in mental status.[34–36] In studies of cultured astrocytes, inflammatory cytokines induced cell swelling.[37] Lipopolysaccharide, a compound found on the bacterial cell wall, has also been shown to enhance ammonia-induced changes in cerebral hemodynamics.[38] In a clinical study of patients with cirrhosis, neuropsychological dysfunction found in the presence of hyperammonemia and SIRS improved after resolution of SIRS.[39] Although the exact mechanisms by which inflammation contributes to the development of HE have not been elucidated, possibilities include cytokine-mediated changes in BBB permeability, altered glutamate uptake by astrocytes, and altered expression of GABA receptors.[39]

Manganese Toxicity

In healthy patients, manganese is cleared by the liver and excreted into the bile. In cirrhotic patients, the elimination of manganese is decreased secondary to portosystemic shunting, which results in increased blood manganese levels and increased cerebral manganese deposition. However, the role of manganese in HE remains unclear. In vitro studies revealed that manganese exposure may cause Alzheimer type II astrocytosis and altered expression of astrocyte proteins.[40] In addition, manganese reduces astrocyte glutamate uptake, alters glutamatergic neurotransmission, and impairs cerebral energy metabolism.[41] Manganese may also cause increased expression of PTBR binding sites,[42] and it has been shown to be involved in the development of hepatic parkinsonism.[43] Cerebral magnetic resonance imaging (MRI) in cirrhotic patients has shown changes likely due to the deposition of manganese.[44–46] Increased manganese content in the brain of cirrhotic patients who died of hepatic coma was noted particularly in the pallidum, putamen, and caudate nucleus.[46] This is in accordance with the significant correlation noted between the ratio of globus pallidus signal intensity compared with frontal subcortical white matter signal intensity and blood manganese levels.[43,44]

CLINICAL FEATURES
HE in Chronic Liver Disease

An acute episode of HE typically manifests as a combination of impaired mental status and neuromuscular dysfunction occurring over a period of hours to days. Altered consciousness includes a variety of symptoms ranging from changes in personality and sleep disturbance to disorientation, stupor, and coma.[47] Evaluation of the severity of HE is based on the West Haven criteria of altered mental status (**Table 1**).[1] A common finding on physical examination is asterixis, which is an inability to maintain position. Asterixis is most commonly tested by having the patient outstretch his or her arms and hold them in dorsiflexion. Asterixis may also be elicited with tongue protrusion, dorsiflexion of the foot, or having the patient grasp the examiner's fingers.[48] As HE advances, asterixis occurs less often and in the state of HE-induced coma it disappears. In a comatose state, the patient may have other physical signs such as hypertonia, extensor plantar responses, or exaggeration of deep tendon reflexes that may progress to generalized flaccidity and hypotonia. As HE resolves, the patient often recovers without permanent neurologic deficits.

Patients with chronic HE (types B and C) have either episodic or persistent symptoms. In those with recurrent episodes, HE may be triggered by noncompliance to

Table 1
West Haven criteria of altered mental status in hepatic encephalopathy[1]

Grade	Consciousness	Intellect and Behavior	Neurologic Findings
0	Normal	Normal	Normal; impaired psychomotor testing
1	Mild lack of awareness	Shortened attention span; impaired addition or subtraction	Mild asterixis or tremor
2	Lethargic	Disoriented; inappropriate behavior	Obvious asterixis; slurred speech
3	Somnolent but arousable	Gross disorientation; bizarre behavior	Muscular rigidity and clonus; hyperreflexia
4	Coma	Coma	Decerebrate posturing

therapy or by a precipitating factor such as infection, gastrointestinal bleeding, or constipation. Between episodes, the patient's mental status may be normal. Those with persistent HE have symptoms that do not reverse despite appropriate medical treatment. These abnormalities may be mild, such as increased muscle tone, dysarthria, or apraxia, or severe, such as dementia, parkinsonism, or myelopathy. Hepatic dementia commonly causes symptoms of dysarthria, apraxia, and decreased concentration. Parkinsonism resembles the clinical findings of Parkinson disease, however there is often a lack of resting tremor.[49] Hepatic myelopathy typically manifests as spastic paraparesis, hyperreflexia, and extensor plantar response.[50]

Minimal Hepatic Encephalopathy

Minimal hepatic encephalopathy (MHE) is a milder form of cognitive impairment that is often undetectable by clinical evaluation.[1] Symptoms and diagnostic criteria for this condition have not been well defined, which further leads to lack of diagnosis in many patients. Although MHE is without clinically overt symptoms, patients often have mild impairment in cognitive function leading to diminished capacity to work or drive.[51] Diagnosis of MHE is based on a combination of history and physical examination and performance on neuropsychological testing. Other etiologies of cognitive impairment should be excluded such as metabolic disturbances and structural brain lesions.

There is no consensus regarding the selection of patients for neuropsychological testing to determine MHE or the type of testing needed to establish a diagnosis. Guidelines provided by the working party at the 11th WCOG suggest using the number connection test (A and B), the digit symbol test, and the block design test, because of their high specificity for MHE.[1,52] The number connection tests, also called Trailmaking A and B, evaluate concentration, mental tracking, and visuomotor skills. The digit symbol test evaluates concentration and mental and motor speed. The block design test studies visuospatial function by asking the patient to copy the design of an object using blocks.[53] On the basis of such testing, it has been demonstrated that the deficits of MHE are mainly in the attention and visuospatial domains.[54] Memory deficits seem to involve primarily short-term memory, and this may be actually caused by diminished attention.[49,52,55] Oral and written verbal skills seem to remain intact. Another less cumbersome diagnostic study available to evaluate MHE is critical flicker frequency (CFF). This tool measures the visual discrimination threshold rate at which light from an intermittent or fluctuating source begins to be seen as continuous or fused. Two large studies have shown this test to correlate significantly with neuropsychological impairment in patients with MHE diagnosed using psychometric testing.[56,57] However, further validation is required.

Neuroimaging studies have been used to evaluate structural abnormalities in MHE. SPECT studies have shown correlation with changes in cerebral blood flow and deficits in memory, cognition, and psychomotor speed as assessed by neuropsychological testing.[58-60] MRI has revealed alterations of the basal ganglia and globus pallidus hyperintensity on T1-weighted images, possibly from manganese deposition.[60-62] Magnetic resonance spectroscopy (MRS) demonstrated an increase in glutamine and glutamate concentration in patients with MHE, most prominently in the basal ganglia.[63] Diffusion-weighted imaging (DWI) has shown that mean diffusivity, an indicator of cerebral edema, is significantly higher in patients with MHE.[64]

MHE can affect quality of life by diminishing a patient's capacity to execute daily functions, such as performance at work or driving. One study, which measured concurrent motor and psychomotor deficits against the physical requirements of the job, implied that 60% of "blue collar" workers were unfit to work, whereas 20% of "white collar" workers were unfit to work.[51] This study also evaluated the effect of MHE on driving. By using neuropsychological tests, a driving simulator, and on-the-road testing, the investigators found that patients with MHE do not demonstrate impaired driving ability.[51] In another study using similar testing and a driving simulator, approximately 44% of patients with MHE were found to be unfit to drive.[65] Additional studies have demonstrated that patients with MHE drive at slower speeds, have more collisions, and have difficulty with following road signs and traffic rules.[66] Although no consensus is available on whether to allow patients with MHE to drive, it is advisable to assess a patient's capacity with neuropsychological testing or driving simulation before permitting them to drive.

Transjugular Intrahepatic Portosystemic Shunt

One of the main drawbacks of transjugular intrahepatic portosystemic shunt (TIPS) is the development of HE; the incidence of new or worsening HE after TIPS is reported to be around 30% to 35%.[67-69] Past history of encephalopathy[67] and increasing age[68] have been identified as important risk factors in post-TIPS HE. It has previously been suggested that post-TIPS HE is associated with a lower hepatic-venous pressure gradient,[70] implying that effective portal decompression increases the risk of HE. Others factors associated with an increased risk of post-TIPS HE include female sex and a cause other than alcoholic liver disease.[69]

Post-TIPS HE tends to occur soon after TIPS insertion. It has been suggested that this temporal relationship relates to cerebral adaptation to gut-derived neurotoxins, which may occur within a few months of the TIPS procedure.[71] Usually, the HE will resolve with conservative therapy. Less frequently, more persistent encephalopathy develops, either because of subsequent progression of the underlying liver disease or in association with preterminal illness. In certain cases, radiologic intervention can be undertaken to resolve refractory HE. However, this occurs at the expense of a predictable recurrence of portal hypertension, which can be problematic especially in the presence of progressive underlying liver disease. In a recent study, post-TIPS HE resistant to conventional treatment and requiring shunt modification was present in 38 of 733 patients.[72]

MANAGEMENT AND THERAPY
Correction of Precipitating Factors

Proper management of HE requires identification and treatment of precipitating factors, as well as exclusion of other causes of altered mental status. Multiple precipitating factors may be present. Most commonly the precipitating incident is either medical noncompliance or infection. Additional precipitating factors include excess protein load by way of gastrointestinal bleeding or dietary intake, centrally acting medications such as sedatives, analgesics, or antidepressants, and fluid/electrolyte imbalance such as hyponatremia, hypokalemia, or dehydration.[73,74] A list of precipitating factors is included in **Box 1**. The causal factor should be actively searched for and identified. The patient should be asked about compliance with treatment, symptoms indicating infection, or use of sedative or analgesic medications. If the patient is unable to give an accurate history, this information should be sought from family members or caretakers.

Laboratory and radiologic investigations can also help in identifying precipitating factors. Dehydration is easily corrected and can be detected through physical signs such as dry mucous membranes, skin tenting, or orthostatic hypotension, as well as laboratory findings of elevated serum creatinine or hemoconcentration. Dehydration is reversed by discontinuation of diuretics and administration of intravenous fluids. Gastrointestinal bleeding can be identified through changes in hemoglobin or elevation of blood urea nitrogen. The patient's current hemoglobin level should always be compared with previous hemoglobin levels, as the patient may be anemic at baseline. If infection is suspected or the patient has clinical evidence of ascites, a paracentesis should be performed with analysis of cell count, gram stain, and culture to evaluate for spontaneous bacterial peritonitis. Additional investigations for infection should be performed with blood cultures, urinalysis, or chest radiographs. Broadspectrum antibiotics should be initiated after obtaining cultures if infection is suspected, especially in patients with stage III or IV HE. Hypokalemia can be corrected with oral or intravenous potassium. Severe hyponatremia, particularly serum sodium

---

Box 1
Hepatic encephalopathy–precipitating factors

Noncompliance to therapy

Dehydration

Gastrointestinal bleeding

Infections

Constipation

Excessive dietary protein

Medications (narcotics, benzodiazepines)

Hyponatremia

Hypokalemia

Renal failure

Surgery

Transjugular intrahepatic portosystemic shunt

Hepatocellular carcinoma

less than 120 mEq/L, should be addressed with appropriate free-water restriction. Vasopressin receptor antagonists may be considered for symptomatic patients with severe hyponatremia.[75] HE precipitated by dietary protein intake or use of sedatives often resolves gradually with supportive care. For patients in whom a precipitating factor has not been identified with history and standard laboratory investigations, the authors recommend ultrasonography with venous Doppler to evaluate for hepatocellular carcinoma or portal vein thrombosis, both of which may worsen portosystemic shunting.

Pharmacologic Therapy

Nonabsorbable disaccharides

The nonabsorbable disaccharides include lactulose and lactitol. Their role in the treatment of HE is to reduce the intestinal production and absorption of ammonia, which is achieved through a laxative effect, movement of ammonia from the portal circulation into the colon, and interference with the uptake of glutamine by the intestinal mucosa and its subsequent metabolism to ammonia.[76,77] Lactulose is generally prescribed as syrup with typical dosages of 15 to 30 mL given 2 to 4 times a day and titrated so the patient has 3 to 5 bowel movements daily. Lactulose can also be given rectally, which is preferable if the patient is unable to take medications orally.[78] Patients may develop aversion to its taste or have symptoms of flatulence or abdominal discomfort. Lactitol, dispensed as a crystalline powder, is generally better tolerated and is as efficacious as lactulose.[79,80] There is no equivalence between the effective doses of lactulose and lactitol.

Nonabsorbable disaccharides are considered the first-line therapy for treatment of acute HE, and improvement in symptoms occurs in 67% to 87%. A placebo-controlled trial showed that lactulose significantly improves cognitive function and health-related quality of life in patients with MHE.[81] In a systematic review, the efficacy of nonabsorbable disaccharides was compared with either no intervention or placebo; the overall treatment effect was modest but statistically significant, with a relative risk of no improvement ranging from 0.62 to 0.92.[82] The review also assessed the comparative efficacy of nonabsorbable disaccharides and antibiotics; patients taking a nonabsorbable disaccharide had a significantly greater risk of no improvement with a relative risk of 1.24.[82]

Antibiotics

Neomycin and metronidazole

Antibiotics such as neomycin or metronidazole reduce intestinal ammonia production by acting against urease-producing bacteria. However, there are limited data regarding the efficacy of these medications. A randomized, controlled study of neomycin 6 g/d versus placebo in 39 patients with acute HE demonstrated no significant difference in time to improvement of symptoms.[83] Two additional studies found no significant difference between lactulose and neomycin.[84,85] A study of 80 patients that evaluated a combination of neomycin and lactulose demonstrated no benefit against placebo.[86] Another trial compared the efficacy of metronidazole with neomycin and showed that both treatments improved mental state and EEG measurements although neither treatment improved mean blood ammonia levels.[87] Side effects of neomycin include intestinal malabsorption, nephrotoxicity, and ototoxicity.[88,89] Metronidazole can cause metallic taste and peripheral neuropathy.[90]

Rifaximin

Rifaximin is an oral antibiotic with minimal side effects and no reported drug interactions. Multiple studies have evaluated its safety and efficacy in patients with stage 1 to 3 HE.[91–95] One prospective study examined a dose-response effect of rifaximin ranging from 600 mg/d to 2400 mg/d administered for 7 days. Significant improvement was observed with dosages of 1200 or 2400 mg/d but not with 600 mg/d.[91] Another randomized, double-blind controlled study compared rifaximin 1200 mg/d to neomycin 3 g/d.[92] After 21 days of treatment, symptoms and blood ammonia levels were significantly reduced in both groups, although reduction in blood ammonia levels was significantly greater with rifaximin. In addition, patients treated with neomycin were more likely to develop adverse side effects such as an increased serum creatinine level, nausea, vomiting, and abdominal pain.

Rifaximin has also been compared with nonabsorbable disaccharides.[93,96] A study of rifaximin 1200 mg/d versus lactitol 60 g/d administered for 5 to 10 days showed approximately 80% symptomatic improvement in both groups.[93] Another trial demonstrated significantly greater improvement in blood ammonia concentrations, EEG results, and mental status with rifaximin 1200 mg/d compared with lactulose 60 g/d.[97] A study of 40 patients with randomization to rifaximin 1200 mg/d or lactulose 120 g/d for the first 2 weeks of each month for 90 days showed improved mental status compared with baseline in both groups; however, improvement was significantly greater with rifaximin than with lactulose. Furthermore, no adverse effects were reported with rifaximin, whereas symptoms of abdominal pain and nausea developed among 75% of patients taking lactulose.[96] The conclusion from these studies is that rifaximin and nonabsorbable disaccharides reduce blood ammonia levels and improve symptoms, but rifaximin has demonstrated earlier improvement and fewer side effects.

Zinc

Zinc is an essential trace element that plays an important role in the regulation of protein and nitrogen metabolism. Zinc deficiency impairs the activity of urea cycle enzymes and glutamine synthetase.[98–100] Zinc deficiency has been implicated in the pathogenesis of HE as diminished serum zinc levels and their inverse correlation with blood ammonia levels were noted in such patients.[101,102] Zinc supplementation in the treatment of HE is based on a small number of controlled studies that provided inconsistent results regarding efficacy, types and doses of zinc used, and duration of therapy. A double-blind, randomized, placebo-controlled study of zinc acetate 600 mg/d for 7 days demonstrated improved mental status that was associated with increase in serum zinc levels.[144] In a randomized trial comparing zinc sulfate or zinc histidine to placebo, an improvement occurred in HE after 3 months of treatment. In another study, after 3 months of supplementation with 600 mg zinc sulfate daily, there was normalization of serum zinc levels and improvement in neuropsychiatric testing.[103] However, other studies have found minimal change in mental status after zinc supplementation despite an increase in zinc levels and reduction in blood ammonia levels.[104]

Other Therapies

Sodium benzoate

Sodium benzoate may be beneficial in the treatment of HE by increasing urinary excretion of ammonia.[105] However, there are limited data supporting its use. One study compared sodium benzoate with lactulose in patients with acute HE and found improved mental status in 80% and 81% of patients, respectively. Both groups had similar incidence of adverse events.[106]

Dopamine agonists

Although altered dopaminergic transmission has been implicated in the pathogenesis of HE, there is little evidence regarding the benefit of dopaminergic agonists in its therapy.[107,108]

Benzodiazepine receptor antagonists

The benzodiazepine receptor antagonist flumazenil has been evaluated in the treatment of HE. One study compared intravenous flumazenil 2 mg (n = 11) to placebo (n = 10) among cirrhotic patients in hepatic coma. It showed improvement in neurologic symptoms in 6 patients treated with flumazenil compared with none with placebo.[109] In another larger study of cirrhotic patients, intravenous flumazenil (n = 265) was compared with placebo (n = 262).[110] The intervention group showed improvement in neurologic scores in 18% of patients with stage 3 HE and 15% of those with stage 4 HE, as opposed to 4% and 3% of placebo-treated patients, respectively. Flumazenil has also been evaluated in the treatment of mild HE.[111] The study demonstrated significant improvement in HE stage and number connection test score compared with placebo.

Ornithine, levocarnitine, and acarbose

L-Ornithine-L-aspartate has been demonstrated to reduce blood ammonia levels by providing substrates for the intracellular conversion of ammonia to urea and glutamine.[107] Results from controlled trials suggest that ornithine aspartate confers therapeutic benefit to patients with chronic, mild to moderate HE as shown by improvement in blood ammonia concentration, HE grade, and PSE index.[112,113]

Levocarnitine has been suggested to lower blood ammonia levels by enhancing metabolic energy production.[105] The findings from clinical studies have been equivocal, with 1 study of 150 patients with mild to moderate HE showing significant improvement in mental status and reduction in blood ammonia levels compared with placebo.[114] However, another study showed no significant changes regarding ammonia levels.[115]

Acarbose is a medication used primarily in the treatment of diabetes mellitus. Although the exact mechanism in HE is unknown, it may be related to inhibition of α-glucosidase in the intestinal brush border. One study using acarbose 150 to 300 mg/d demonstrated significant lowering of blood ammonia levels and improvement in number connection test scores compared with placebo.[116] However, acarbose was associated with adverse side effects including abdominal pain, flatulence, and diarrhea.

Probiotics

Probiotics are defined as live microbiologic dietary supplements that have beneficial effects on the host beyond their nutritive value. The mechanism of action of probiotics in HE is postulated to be the deprivation of substrates for potentially pathogenic bacteria, and the provision of fermentation end products for potentially beneficial bacteria.[117,118] Stool studies from patients with MHE showed that probiotic supplementation was associated with a decrease in *Escherichia coli*, *Fusobacterium,* and staphylococci and an increase in nonurease-producing *Lactobacillus*.[119] Several clinical studies have evaluated the use of probiotics in the management of MHE. A randomized study of *Enterococcus faecium* SF68 and lactulose showed better efficacy of *E. faecium* SF68 in reducing blood ammonia levels and improvement in neurocognitive testing.[120] An additional study demonstrated improvement in MHE in patients treated with Synbiotic 2000, a combination of probiotic and fiber.[119] Another study compared *Bifidobacterium longum* with fructo-oligosaccharide with placebo and found significant improvement in neuropsychological test results and blood ammonia levels.[121] A recent study examined the use of probiotic yogurt in the management of MHE.[122] The study found a significantly higher proportion of patients taking yogurt reversed MHE by neuropsychological testing compared with no treatment. Given the reported efficacy of probiotics and their lack of side effects, they may be a useful alternative in the management of MHE.

Nutrition

Protein-calorie malnutrition has been observed in all stages of liver disease, particularly end-stage liver disease. Factors that contribute to this nutritional deficit include diminished oral intake, hypermetabolic state, bacterial overgrowth from impaired small-bowel motility, and gastrointestinal protein loss.[123] Guidelines published by the European Society for Clinical Nutrition and Metabolism (ESPEN) recommended that patients with cirrhosis should have an energy intake of 35 to 40 kcal/kg body weight per day and a protein intake of 1.2 to 1.5 g/kg body weight per day.[124] If oral intake is inadequate, additional oral nutritional supplements or tube feeding should be commenced. The belief among certain clinicians is to restrict protein in cirrhotic patients, especially those with HE. However, one randomized controlled trial comparing high (1.2 g/kg/d) with low (0.5 g/kg/d) protein diets showed that restricting protein intake during encephalopathy had no beneficial effect.[125] This study also reported that a low protein diet led to increased protein catabolism. Another trial found that increased protein intake was associated with efficient protein retention but did not result in HE.[126]

Branched-chain amino acids (BCAAs) may have a therapeutic role in the treatment of HE. They have been shown to improve regional cerebral blood flow in patients with cirrhosis.[127] In a large, multicenter, randomized trial of patients with cirrhosis, BCAAs improved combined rate of death and progression to liver failure.[128] A Cochrane review of 11 randomized trials (556 patients) confirmed that BCAAs significantly increased the number of patients improving from HE.[129] In general, BCAAs were more effective if given enterally than intravenously.

Liver Support Devices

Artificial liver support systems are designed to purify blood by removing protein-bound and water-soluble toxins without providing liver synthetic functions. Currently available systems are based on albumin dialysis or plasma separation and filtration. Bioartificial liver support (BAL) refers to systems that use viable hepatocytes as components of an extracorporeal device connected to the patient's circulation, and therefore have the potential to provide liver function. They consist of a bioreactor containing hepatocytes with or without a blood purification device.

Studies examining the role of extracorporeal liver support devices have consistently demonstrated an improvement in HE. Although several of these studies were performed in a randomized, controlled fashion, the duration of application was short, usually for a period of a few days. Therefore, no conclusions could be made regarding long-term efficacy and effect on survival.[130–132] The mechanism by which liver support devices improve HE may be related to reduction in blood ammonia levels. However, the findings have been contradictory, and their effect may also be attributed to clearance of aromatic amino acids and endogenous benzodiazepines.[130,133–138]

SUMMARY

HE encompasses a spectrum of neuropsychiatric symptoms and signs among patients with liver failure. Severe HE portends poor outcome and is considered an indication for liver transplantation. In patients with cirrhosis and portosystemic shunting, HE causes functional impairment and significant morbidity. Several factors (particularly ammonia) have been implicated in its pathogenesis. Treatment is directed at the correction of precipitating factors such as sepsis, gastrointestinal bleeding, medications, and fluid and electrolyte imbalance. The mainstay of pharmacologic management includes nonabsorbable disaccharides, principally lactulose, and antibiotics such as neomycin, metronidazole, and rifaximin. The role of liver support devices remains to be established.

REFERENCES

1. Ferenci P, Lockwood A, Mullen K, et al. Hepatic encephalopathy—definition, nomenclature, diagnosis, and quantification: final report of the working party at the 11th World Congresses of Gastroenterology, Vienna, 1998. Hepatology 2002;35:716–21.
2. Munoz SJ. Hepatic encephalopathy. Med Clin North Am 2008;92:795–812, viii.
3. Haussinger D, Schliess F. Pathogenetic mechanisms of hepatic encephalopathy. Gut 2008;57:1156–65.
4. Gerber T, Schomerus H. Hepatic encephalopathy in liver cirrhosis: pathogenesis, diagnosis and management. Drugs 2000;60:1353–70.
5. Butterworth RF. Complications of cirrhosis III. Hepatic encephalopathy. J Hepatol 2000;32:171–80.
6. Diemer NH. Number of Purkinje cells and Bergmann astrocytes in rats with CCl_4-induced liver disease. Acta Neurol Scand 1977;55:1–15.
7. Pilbeam CM, Anderson RM, Bhathal PS. The brain in experimental portal-systemic encephalopathy. I. Morphological changes in three animal models. J Pathol 1983;140:331–45.
8. Albrecht J, Norenberg MD. Glutamine: a Trojan horse in ammonia neurotoxicity. Hepatology 2006;44:788–94.
9. Corbalan R, Hernandez-Viadel M, Llansola M, et al. Chronic hyperammonemia alters protein phosphorylation and glutamate receptor-associated signal transduction in brain. Neurochem Int 2002;41:103–8.
10. Schliess F, Gorg B, Fischer R, et al. Ammonia induces MK-801-sensitive nitration and phosphorylation of protein tyrosine residues in rat astrocytes. FASEB J 2002;16:739–41.
11. Schliess F, Foster N, Gorg B, et al. Hypoosmotic swelling increases protein tyrosine nitration in cultured rat astrocytes. Glia 2004;47:21–9.
12. Murthy CR, Rama Rao KV, Bai G, et al. Ammonia-induced production of free radicals in primary cultures of rat astrocytes. J Neurosci Res 2001;66:282–8.
13. Jayakumar AR, Rama Rao KV, Schousboe A, et al. Glutamine-induced free radical production in cultured astrocytes. Glia 2004;46:296–301.
14. Rama Rao KV, Chen M, Simard JM, et al. Suppression of ammonia-induced astrocyte swelling by cyclosporin A. J Neurosci Res 2003;74:891–7.
15. Rama Rao KV, Norenberg MD. Aquaporin-4 in hepatic encephalopathy. Metab Brain Dis 2007;22:265–75.
16. Chepkova AN, Sergeeva OA, Haas HL. Taurine rescues hippocampal long-term potentiation from ammonia-induced impairment. Neurobiol Dis 2006;23:512–21.

17. Jalan R, Olde Damink SW, Lui HF, et al. Oral amino acid load mimicking hemo-globin results in reduced regional cerebral perfusion and deterioration in memory tests in patients with cirrhosis of the liver. Metab Brain Dis 2003;18: 37–49.

18. Lockwood AH, Yap EW, Wong WH. Cerebral ammonia metabolism in patients with severe liver disease and minimal hepatic encephalopathy. J Cereb Blood Flow Metab 1991;11:337–41.

19. Weissenborn K, Bokemeyer M, Ahl B, et al. Functional imaging of the brain in patients with liver cirrhosis. Metab Brain Dis 2004;19:269–80.

20. Bansky G, Meier PS, Ziegler WH, et al. Reversal of hepatic coma by benzodiaz-epine antagonists (Ro 15-1788) [letter]. Lancet 1985;1:1324–5.

21. Scollo-Lavizzari G, Steinmann E. Reversal of hepatic coma by benzodiazepine antagonist (Ro 15-1788) [letter]. Lancet 1985;1:1324.

22. Lighthouse J, Naito Y, Helmy A, et al. Endotoxinemia and benzodiazepine-like substances in compensated cirrhotic patients: a randomized study comparing the effect of rifaximine alone and in association with a symbiotic preparation. Hepatol Res 2004;28:155–60.

23. Zeneroli ML, Venturini I, Corsi L, et al. Benzodiazepine-like compounds in the plasma of patients with fulminant hepatic failure. Scand J Gastroenterol 1998; 33:310–3.

24. Zeneroli ML, Venturini I, Stefanelli S, et al. Antibacterial activity of rifaximin reduces the levels of benzodiazepine-like compounds in patients with liver cirrhosis. Pharmacol Res 1997;35:557–60.

25. Basile AS, Jones EA. The involvement of benzodiazepine receptor ligands in hepatic encephalopathy. Hepatology 1994;20:541–3.

26. Stewart CA, Reivich M, Lucey MR, et al. Neuroimaging in hepatic encephalop-athy. Clin Gastroenterol Hepatol 2005;3:197–207.

27. Cagnin A, Taylor-Robinson SD, Forton DM, et al. In vivo imaging of cerebral "peripheral benzodiazepine binding sites" in patients with hepatic encephalop-athy. Gut 2006;55:547–53.

28. Ahboucha S, Layrargues GP, Mamer O, et al. Increased brain concentrations of a neuroinhibitory steroid in human hepatic encephalopathy. Ann Neurol 2005;58: 169–70.

29. Baraldi M, Zeneroli ML, Ventura E, et al. Supersensitivity of benzodiazepine receptors in hepatic encephalopathy due to fulminant hepatic failure in the rat: reversal by a benzodiazepine antagonist. Clin Sci (Lond) 1984;67:167–75.

30. Schafer DF, Fowler JM, Munson PJ, et al. Gamma-aminobutyric acid and benzo-diazepine receptors in an animal model of fulminant hepatic failure. J Lab Clin Med 1983;102:870–80.

31. Butterworth RF, Lavoie J, Giguere JF, et al. Affinities and densities of high-affinity [^{3}H]muscimol (GABA-A) binding sites and of central benzodiazepine receptors are unchanged in autopsied brain tissue from cirrhotic patients with hepatic encephalopathy. Hepatology 1988;8:1084–8.

32. Ahboucha S, Desjardins P, Chatauret N, et al. Normal coupling of brain benzo-diazepine and neurosteroid modulatory sites on the GABA-A receptor complex in human hepatic encephalopathy. Neurochem Int 2003;43:551–6.

33. Dodd PR, Thomas GJ, Harper CG, et al. Amino acid neurotransmitter receptor changes in cerebral cortex in alcoholism: effect of cirrhosis of the liver. J Neuro-chem 1992;59:1506–15.

34. Blei AT. Infection, inflammation and hepatic encephalopathy, synergism rede-fined. J Hepatol 2004;40:327–30.

35. Rolando N, Wade J, Davalos M, et al. The systemic inflammatory response syndrome in acute liver failure. Hepatology 2000;32:734–9.
36. Vaquero J, Polson J, Chung C, et al. Infection and the progression of hepatic encephalopathy in acute liver failure. Gastroenterology 2003;125:755–64.
37. Haussinger D, Schliess F. Astrocyte swelling and protein tyrosine nitration in hepatic encephalopathy. Neurochem Int 2005;47:64–70.
38. Pedersen HR, Ring-Larsen H, Olsen NV, et al. Hyperammonemia acts synergistically with lipopolysaccharide in inducing changes in cerebral hemodynamics in rats anaesthetised with pentobarbital. J Hepatol 2007;47:245–52.
39. Shawcross DL, Davies NA, Williams R, et al. Systemic inflammatory response exacerbates the neuropsychological effects of induced hyperammonemia in cirrhosis. J Hepatol 2004;40:247–54.
40. Hazell AS. Astrocytes and manganese neurotoxicity. Neurochem Int 2002;41: 271–7.
41. Hazell AS, Desjardins P, Butterworth RF. Increased expression of glyceraldehyde-3-phosphate dehydrogenase in cultured astrocytes following exposure to manganese. Neurochem Int 1999;35:11–7.
42. Hazell AS, Desjardins P, Butterworth RF. Chronic exposure of rat primary astrocyte cultures to manganese results in increased binding sites for the 'peripheral-type' benzodiazepine receptor ligand ^{3}H-PK 11195. Neurosci Lett 1999; 271:5–8.
43. Krieger D, Krieger S, Jansen O, et al. Manganese and chronic hepatic encephalopathy. Lancet 1995;346:270–4.
44. Spahr L, Butterworth RF, Fontaine S, et al. Increased blood manganese in cirrhotic patients: relationship to pallidal magnetic resonance signal hyperintensity and neurological symptoms. Hepatology 1996;24:1116–20.
45. Weissenborn K, Ehrenheim C, Hori A, et al. Pallidal lesions in patients with liver cirrhosis: clinical and MRI evaluation. Metab Brain Dis 1995;10:219–31.
46. Rose C, Butterworth RF, Zayed J, et al. Manganese deposition in basal ganglia structures results from both portal-systemic shunting and liver dysfunction. Gastroenterology 1999;117:640–4.
47. Adams RD, Foley JM. The neurological disorder associated with liver disease. Res Publ Assoc Res Nerv Ment Dis 1953;32:198–237.
48. Timmermann L, Gross J, Butz M, et al. Mini-asterixis in hepatic encephalopathy induced by pathologic thalamo-motor-cortical coupling. Neurology 2003;61: 689–92.
49. Joebges EM, Heidemann M, Schimke N, et al. Bradykinesia in minimal hepatic encephalopathy is due to disturbances in movement initiation. J Hepatol 2003; 38:273–80.
50. Mendoza G, Marti-Fabregas J, Kulisevsky J, et al. Hepatic myelopathy: a rare complication of portacaval shunt. Eur Neurol 1994;34:209–12.
51. Schomerus H, Hamster W. Quality of life in cirrhotics with minimal hepatic encephalopathy. Metab Brain Dis 2001;16:37–41.
52. Weissenborn K, Ennen JC, Schomerus H, et al. Neuropsychological characterization of hepatic encephalopathy. J Hepatol 2001;34:768–73.
53. Howieson DB, Lezak MD. The neuropsychological evaluation. In: Yudofsky SC, Hales RE, editors. Textbook of neuropsychiatry and clinical neurosciences. Washington, DC: American Psychiatric Publishing; 2002.
54. McCrea M, Cordoba J, Vessey G, et al. Neuropsychological characterization and detection of subclinical hepatic encephalopathy. Arch Neurol 1996;53: 758–63.

55. Weissenborn K, Bokemeyer M, Krause J, et al. Neurological and neuropsychiatric syndromes associated with liver disease. AIDS 2005;3(Suppl 19):S93–8.

56. Romero-Gomez M, Cordoba J, Jover R, et al. Value of the critical flicker frequency in patients with minimal hepatic encephalopathy. Hepatology 2007; 45:879–85.

57. Sharma P, Sharma BC, Puri V, et al. Critical flicker frequency: diagnostic tool for minimal hepatic encephalopathy. J Hepatol 2007;47:67–73.

58. O'Carroll RE, Hayes PC, Ebmeier KP, et al. Regional cerebral blood flow and cognitive function in patients with chronic liver disease. Lancet 1991;337:1250–3.

59. Trzepacz PT. The neuropathogenesis of delirium. A need to focus our research. Psychosomatics 1994;35:374–91.

60. Catafau AM, Kulisevsky J, Berna L, et al. Relationship between cerebral perfusion in frontal-limbic-basal ganglia circuits and neuropsychologic impairment in patients with subclinical hepatic encephalopathy. J Nucl Med 2000;41:405–10.

61. Morgan MY. Cerebral magnetic resonance imaging in patients with chronic liver disease. Metab Brain Dis 1998;13:273–90.

62. Malecki EA, Devenyi AG, Barron TF, et al. Iron and manganese homeostasis in chronic liver disease: relationship to pallidal T1-weighted magnetic resonance signal hyperintensity. Neurotoxicology 1999;20:647–52.

63. Weissenborn K, Ahl B, Fischer-Wasels D, et al. Correlations between magnetic resonance spectroscopy alterations and cerebral ammonia and glucose metabolism in cirrhotic patients with and without hepatic encephalopathy. Gut 2007;56: 1736–42.

64. Kale RA, Gupta RK, Saraswat VA, et al. Demonstration of interstitial cerebral edema with diffusion tensor MR imaging in type C hepatic encephalopathy. Hepatology 2006;43:698–706.

65. Watanabe A, Tuchida T, Yata Y, et al. Evaluation of neuropsychological function in patients with liver cirrhosis with special reference to their driving ability. Metab Brain Dis 1995;10:239–48.

66. Wein C, Koch H, Popp B, et al. Minimal hepatic encephalopathy impairs fitness to drive. Hepatology 2004;39:739–45.

67. Jalan R, Elton RA, Redhead DN, et al. Analysis of prognostic variables in the prediction of mortality, shunt failure, variceal rebleeding and encephalopathy following the transjugular intrahepatic portosystemic stent-shunt for variceal haemorrhage. J Hepatol 1995;23:123–8.

68. Sanyal AJ, Freedman AM, Shiffman ML, et al. Portosystemic encephalopathy after transjugular intrahepatic portosystemic shunt: results of a prospective controlled study. Hepatology 1994;20:46–55.

69. Somberg KA, Riegler JL, LaBerge JM, et al. Hepatic encephalopathy after transjugular intrahepatic portosystemic shunts: incidence and risk factors. Am J Gastroenterol 1995;90:549–55.

70. Casado M, Bosch J, Garcia-Pagan JC, et al. Clinical events after transjugular intrahepatic portosystemic shunt: correlation with hemodynamic findings. Gastroenterology 1998;114:1296–303.

71. Nolte W, Wiltfang J, Schindler C, et al. Portosystemic hepatic encephalopathy after transjugular intrahepatic portosystemic shunt in patients with cirrhosis: clinical, laboratory, psychometric, and electroencephalographic investigations. Hepatology 1998;28:1215–25.

72. Kochar N, Tripathi D, Ireland H, et al. Transjugular intrahepatic portosystemic stent shunt (TIPSS) modification in the management of post-TIPSS refractory hepatic encephalopathy. Gut 2006;55:1617–23.

73. Phillips GB, Schwartz R, Gabuzda GJ Jr, et al. The syndrome of impending hepatic coma in patients with cirrhosis of the liver given certain nitrogenous substances. N Engl J Med 1952;247:239–46.
74. Schwartz R, Phillips GB, Seegmiller JE, et al. Dietary protein in the genesis of hepatic coma. N Engl J Med 1954;251:685–9.
75. Schrier RW, Gross P, Gheorghiade M, et al. Tolvaptan, a selective oral vaso-pressin V2-receptor antagonist, for hyponatremia. N Engl J Med 2006;355: 2099–112.
76. van Leeuwen PA, van Berlo CL, Soeters PB. New mode of action for lactulose. Lancet 1988;1:55–6.
77. Cordoba J, Minguez B, Vergara M. Treatment of hepatic encephalopathy. Lancet 2005;365:1384–5 [author reply 1385–6].
78. Uribe M, Campollo O, Vargas F, et al. Acidifying enemas (lactitol and lactose) vs. nonacidifying enemas (tap water) to treat acute portal-systemic encephalop-athy: a double-blind, randomized clinical trial. Hepatology 1987;7:639–43.
79. Morgan MY, Hawley KE. Lactitol vs. lactulose in the treatment of acute hepatic encephalopathy in cirrhotic patients: a double-blind, randomized trial. Hepatol-ogy 1987;7:1278–84.
80. Morgan MY, Alonso M, Stanger LC. Lactitol and lactulose for the treatment of subclinical hepatic encephalopathy in cirrhotic patients. A randomised, cross-over study. J Hepatol 1989;8:208–17.
81. Prasad S, Dhiman RK, Duseja A, et al. Lactulose improves cognitive functions and health-related quality of life in patients with cirrhosis who have minimal hepatic encephalopathy. Hepatology 2007;45:549–59.
82. Als-Nielsen B, Gluud LL, Gluud C. Non-absorbable disaccharides for hepatic encephalopathy: systematic review of randomised trials. BMJ 2004;328:1046.
83. Strauss E, Tramote R, Silva EP, et al. Double-blind randomized clinical trial comparing neomycin and placebo in the treatment of exogenous hepatic encephalopathy. Hepatogastroenterology 1992;39:542–5.
84. Atterbury CE, Maddrey WC, Conn HO. Neomycin-sorbitol and lactulose in the treatment of acute portal-systemic encephalopathy. A controlled, double-blind clinical trial. Am J Dig Dis 1978;23:398–406.
85. Conn HO, Leevy CM, Vlahcevic ZR, et al. Comparison of lactulose and neomycin in the treatment of chronic portal-systemic encephalopathy. A double blind controlled trial. Gastroenterology 1977;72:573–83.
86. Blanc P, Daures JP, Liautard J, et al. [Lactulose-neomycin combination versus placebo in the treatment of acute hepatic encephalopathy. Results of a random-ized controlled trial]. Gastroenterol Clin Biol 1994;18:1063–8 [in French].
87. Morgan MH, Read AE, Speller DC. Treatment of hepatic encephalopathy with metronidazole. Gut 1982;23:1–7.
88. Hawkins RA, Jessy J, Mans AM, et al. Neomycin reduces the intestinal produc-tion of ammonia from glutamine. Adv Exp Med Biol 1994;368:125–34.
89. Green PH, Tall AR. Drugs, alcohol and malabsorption. Am J Med 1979;67: 1066–76.
90. Bustamante J, Rimola A, Ventura PJ, et al. Prognostic significance of hepatic encephalopathy in patients with cirrhosis. J Hepatol 1999;30:890–5.
91. Bass NM, Ahmed A, Johnson L, et al. Rifaximin treatment is beneficial for mild hepatic encephalopathy. Hepatology 2004;40:646A [abstract].
92. Pedretti G, Calzetti C, Missale G, et al. Rifaximin versus neomycin on hyperam-moniemia in chronic portal systemic encephalopathy of cirrhotics. A double-blind, randomized trial. Ital J Gastroenterol 1991;23:175–8.

93. Mas A, Rodes J, Sunyer L, et al. Comparison of rifaximin and lactitol in the treatment of acute hepatic encephalopathy: results of a randomized, double-blind, double-dummy, controlled clinical trial. J Hepatol 2003;38:51–8.

94. Williams R, James OF, Warnes TW, et al. Evaluation of the efficacy and safety of rifaximin in the treatment of hepatic encephalopathy: a double-blind, randomized, dose-finding multi-centre study. Eur J Gastroenterol Hepatol 2000;12: 203–8.

95. Bucci L, Palmieri GC. Double-blind, double-dummy comparison between treatment with rifaximin and lactulose in patients with medium to severe degree hepatic encephalopathy. Curr Med Res Opin 1993;13:109–18.

96. Giacomo F, Francesco A, Michele N, et al. Rifaximin in the treatment of hepatic encephalopathy. Eur J Clin Res 1993;4:57–66.

97. Massa P, Vallerino E, Dodero M. Treatment of hepatic encephalopathy with rifaximin: double blind, double dummy study versus lactulose. Eur J Clin Res 1993;4: 7–18.

98. Rabbani P, Prasad AS. Plasma ammonia and liver ornithine transcarbamoylase activity in zinc-deficient rats. Am J Physiol 1978;235:E203–6.

99. Riggio O, Merli M, Capocaccia L, et al. Zinc supplementation reduces blood ammonia and increases liver ornithine transcarbamylase activity in experimental cirrhosis. Hepatology 1992;16:785–9.

100. Prasad AS, Rabbani P, Abbasii A, et al. Experimental zinc deficiency in humans. Ann Intern Med 1978;89:483–90.

101. Reding P, Duchateau J, Bataille C. Oral zinc supplementation improves hepatic encephalopathy. Results of a randomised controlled trial. Lancet 1984;2:493–5.

102. Grungreiff K, Presser HJ, Franke D, et al. Correlations between zinc, amino acids and ammonia in liver cirrhosis. Z Gastroenterol 1989;27:731–5.

103. Marchesini G, Fabbri A, Bianchi G, et al. Zinc supplementation and amino acid-nitrogen metabolism in patients with advanced cirrhosis. Hepatology 1996;23: 1084–92.

104. Riggio O, Ariosto F, Merli M, et al. Short-term oral zinc supplementation does not improve chronic hepatic encephalopathy. Results of a double-blind crossover trial. Dig Dis Sci 1991;36:1204–8.

105. Abou-Assi S, Vlahcevic ZR. Hepatic encephalopathy. Metabolic consequence of cirrhosis often is reversible. Postgrad Med 2001;109:52–4, 57–60, 63–5 passim.

106. Sushma S, Dasarathy S, Tandon RK, et al. Sodium benzoate in the treatment of acute hepatic encephalopathy: a double-blind randomized trial. Hepatology 1992;16:138–44.

107. Blei AT, Cordoba J. Hepatic encephalopathy. Am J Gastroenterol 2001;96: 1968–76.

108. Uribe M, Farca A, Marquez MA, et al. Treatment of chronic portal systemic encephalopathy with bromocriptine: a double-blind controlled trial. Gastroenterology 1979;76:1347–51.

109. Pomier-Layrargues G, Giguere JF, Lavoie J, et al. Flumazenil in cirrhotic patients in hepatic coma: a randomized double-blind placebo-controlled crossover trial. Hepatology 1994;19:32–7.

110. Barbaro G, Di Lorenzo G, Soldini M, et al. Flumazenil for hepatic encephalopathy grade III and IVa in patients with cirrhosis: an Italian multicenter double-blind, placebo-controlled, cross-over study. Hepatology 1998;28:374–8.

111. Dursun M, Caliskan M, Canoruc F, et al. The efficacy of flumazenil in subclinical to mild hepatic encephalopathic ambulatory patients. A prospective,

randomised, double-blind, placebo-controlled study. Swiss Med Wkly 2003;133: 118–23.

112. Kircheis G, Nilius R, Held C, et al. Therapeutic efficacy of L-ornithine-L-aspartate infusions in patients with cirrhosis and hepatic encephalopathy: results of a placebo-controlled, double-blind study. Hepatology 1997;25:1351–60.

113. Stauch S, Kircheis G, Adler G, et al. Oral L-ornithine-L-aspartate therapy of chronic hepatic encephalopathy: results of a placebo-controlled double-blind study. J Hepatol 1998;28:856–64.

114. Malaguarnera M, Pistone G, Elvira R, et al. Effects of L-carnitine in patients with hepatic encephalopathy. World J Gastroenterol 2005;11:7197–202.

115. del Olmo JA, Castillo M, Rodrigo JM, et al. Effect of L-carnitine upon ammonia tolerance test in cirrhotic patients. Adv Exp Med Biol 1990;272:197–208.

116. Gentile S, Guarino G, Romano M, et al. A randomized controlled trial of acarbose in hepatic encephalopathy. Clin Gastroenterol Hepatol 2005;3:184–91.

117. Solga SF. Probiotics can treat hepatic encephalopathy. Med Hypotheses 2003; 61:307–13.

118. Bongaerts G, Severijnen R, Timmerman H. Effect of antibiotics, prebiotics and probiotics in treatment for hepatic encephalopathy. Med Hypotheses 2005;64: 64–8.

119. Liu Q, Duan ZP, Ha DK, et al. Synbiotic modulation of gut flora: effect on minimal hepatic encephalopathy in patients with cirrhosis. Hepatology 2004;39:1441–9.

120. Loguercio C, Abbiati R, Rinaldi M, et al. Long-term effects of *Enterococcus faecium* SF68 versus lactulose in the treatment of patients with cirrhosis and grade 1-2 hepatic encephalopathy. J Hepatol 1995;23:39–46.

121. Malaguarnera M, Greco F, Barone G, et al. *Bifidobacterium longum* with fructo-oligosaccharide (FOS) treatment in minimal hepatic encephalopathy: a randomized, double-blind, placebo-controlled study. Dig Dis Sci 2007;52:3259–65.

122. Bajaj JS, Saeian K, Christensen KM, et al. Probiotic yogurt for the treatment of minimal hepatic encephalopathy. Am J Gastroenterol 2008;103:1707–15.

123. Charlton M. Branched-chain amino acid enriched supplements as therapy for liver disease. J Nutr 2006;136:295S–8S.

124. Plauth M, Cabre E, Riggio O, et al. ESPEN guidelines on enteral nutrition: liver disease. Clin Nutr 2006;25:285–94.

125. Cordoba J, Lopez-Hellin J, Planas M, et al. Normal protein diet for episodic hepatic encephalopathy: results of a randomized study. J Hepatol 2004;41:38–43.

126. Nielsen K, Kondrup J, Martinsen L, et al. Long-term oral refeeding of patients with cirrhosis of the liver. Br J Nutr 1995;74:557–67.

127. Iwasa M, Matsumura K, Watanabe Y, et al. Improvement of regional cerebral blood flow after treatment with branched-chain amino acid solutions in patients with cirrhosis. Eur J Gastroenterol Hepatol 2003;15:733–7.

128. Muto Y, Sato S, Watanabe A, et al. Effects of oral branched-chain amino acid granules on event-free survival in patients with liver cirrhosis. Clin Gastroenterol Hepatol 2005;3:705–13.

129. Als-Nielsen B, Koretz RL, Kjaergard LL, et al. Branched-chain amino acids for hepatic encephalopathy. Cochrane Database Syst Rev 2003;2:CD001939.

130. Sen S, Davies NA, Mookerjee RP, et al. Pathophysiological effects of albumin dialysis in acute-on-chronic liver failure: a randomized controlled study. Liver Transpl 2004;10:1109–19.

131. Heemann U, Treichel U, Loock J, et al. Albumin dialysis in cirrhosis with superimposed acute liver injury: a prospective, controlled study. Hepatology 2002;36: 949–58.

132. Hassanein TI, Tofteng F, Brown RS Jr, et al. Randomized controlled study of extracorporeal albumin dialysis for hepatic encephalopathy in advanced cirrhosis. Hepatology 2007;46:1853–62.

133. Krisper P, Haditsch B, Stauber R, et al. In vivo quantification of liver dialysis: comparison of albumin dialysis and fractionated plasma separation. J Hepatol 2005;43:451–7.

134. Sorkine P, Ben Abraham R, Szold O, et al. Role of the molecular adsorbent recycling system (MARS) in the treatment of patients with acute exacerbation of chronic liver failure. Crit Care Med 2001;29:1332–6.

135. Stange J, Mitzner SR, Risler T, et al. Molecular adsorbent recycling system (MARS): clinical results of a new membrane-based blood purification system for bioartificial liver support. Artif Organs 1999;23:319–30.

136. Sen S, Rose C, Ytrebo LM, et al. Effect of albumin dialysis on intracranial pressure increase in pigs with acute liver failure: a randomized study. Crit Care Med 2006;34:158–64.

137. Stange J, Mitzner S. A carrier-mediated transport of toxins in a hybrid membrane. Safety barrier between a patients blood and a bioartificial liver. Int J Artif Organs 1996;19:677–91.

138. Mitzner S, Loock J, Peszynski P, et al. Improvement in central nervous system functions during treatment of liver failure with albumin dialysis MARS – a review of clinical, biochemical, and electrophysiological data. Metab Brain Dis 2002;17:463–75.

Portal Hypertension and Variceal Hemorrhage

David A. Sass, MD[a],*, Kapil B. Chopra, MD, DM[b]

KEYWORDS

- Portal hypertension • HVPG • Varices • Band ligation
- Beta blockers • TIPS

Gastroesophageal variceal hemorrhage is perhaps the most devastating portal hypertension-related complication in patients with cirrhosis, occurring in up to 30% of such individuals during the course of their illness.[1] Variceal hemorrhage is associated with substantial morbidity and mortality: up to 20% of initial bleeding episodes are fatal, and as many as 70% of survivors have recurrent bleeding within 1 year after the index hemorrhage.[1,2] Management of patients with gastroesophageal varices includes: (1) prevention of the initial bleeding episode ("primary prophylaxis"), (2) the control of active hemorrhage, and (3) the prevention of recurrent bleeding after a first episode ("secondary prophylaxis"). This review summarizes the pathophysiology, diagnosis, natural history, and body of literature concerning these 3 aspects of the management of variceal hemorrhage. Medical (both pharmacologic and endoscopic), surgical, and radiologic techniques will each be discussed. Ideally, such treatment should be universally effective, safe, easy to administer, widely available, and relatively inexpensive. Unfortunately, none of the existing treatments comes close to being ideal, and the treatment of portal hypertension continues to remain one of the greatest challenges in the management of a patient with cirrhosis.[3]

PORTAL HEMODYNAMICS AND PATHOGENESIS OF VARICES

Varices are portosystemic collaterals formed after preexisting vascular channels have been dilated by portal hypertension. The major sites of collaterals are around the rectum, umbilicus ("caput medusa"), retroperitoneum, and distal esophagus/proximal stomach. Portal hypertension is a clinical syndrome defined by a portal venous pressure gradient exceeding 5 mm Hg. It can arise from any condition interfering with the

[a] Division of Gastroenterology and Hepatology, Drexel University College of Medicine, 216 N. Broad Street, Feinstein Building, Suite 504, MS 1001, Philadelphia, PA 19102, USA
[b] Division of Gastroenterology, Hepatology and Nutrition, University of Pittsburgh School of Medicine, Pittsburgh, PA, USA
* Corresponding author.
E-mail address: dsass@drexelmed.edu (D.A. Sass).

Med Clin N Am 93 (2009) 837–853
doi:10.1016/j.mcna.2009.03.008
0025-7125/09/$ – see front matter © 2009 Elsevier Inc. All rights reserved.

medical.theclinics.com

blood flow at any level within the portal system and can be classified as prehepatic, intrahepatic, or posthepatic (**Box 1**). Cirrhosis is the most common cause of portal hypertension in the Western world, accounting for about 90% of cases, while schistosomiasis is the leading cause in many other countries.

In cirrhosis, portal pressure increases initially as a consequence of an increased resistance to flow because of an architectural distortion of the liver secondary to fibrous tissue and regenerative nodules. Despite the formation of portosystemic collaterals, portal hypertension persists, as there is also an increase in portal venous inflow that results from splanchnic arteriolar vasodilation. As in any other vessel, the pressure within the portal vein is determined by the product of blood flow and resistance as defined by Ohm's law: P(pressure) = Q(blood flow) × R(resistance).

The hallmark of portal hypertension is a pathologic increase in the pressure gradient between the portal vein and inferior vena cava: the HVPG. The HVPG is the difference between the wedged hepatic vein pressures (WHVP), a marker of sinusoidal pressure, and the FHVP.[4]

$$HVPG = WHVP - FHVP$$

The FHVP is subtracted from the WHVP to correct for intra-abdominal pressure and provide an accurate measure of the portal vein pressure.

NATURAL HISTORY OF VARICES AND PREDICTORS OF HEMORRHAGE

Varices do not form at an HVPG less than 12 mm Hg.[5,6] Although a threshold portal pressure of 12 mm Hg is required for the development of varices, once varices develop, the risk of rupture is largely determined by the variceal-wall tension (T),

---

Box 1
Causes of portal hypertension

Prehepatic portal hypertension (normal wedged hepatic venous pressure (WHVP) and free hepatic venous pressure (FHVP) with normal hepatic venous pressure gradient (HVPG)):

  Portal vein thrombosis

  Splenic vein thrombosis

  Congenital stenosis of portal vein

  Arteriovenous fistula

Intrahepatic portal hypertension (increased WHVP, normal FHVP, increased HVPG):

  Presinusoidal: Primary biliary cirrhosis

  Sinusoidal: cirrhosis, infiltrative liver diseases, idiopathic portal hypertension, congenital hepatic fibrosis, nodular regenerative hyperplasia, and polycystic liver disease

  Postsinusoidal: venoocclusive disease

Posthepatic portal hypertension (increased WHVP and FHVP with normal HVPG):

  Budd-Chiari syndrome

  IVC webs, thrombosis

  Congestive heart failure

  Constrictive pericarditis

  Tricuspid valve diseases

which, according to Frank's modification of Laplace's law ($T = P \times R/W$) is a function of the transmural pressure (P), the radius (R) of the vessel, and the thickness of the vessel wall (W).[7] P is directly related to the HVPG; therefore a reduction in HVPG should lead to a decrease in T and then to a decrease in the risk for rupture. This has been confirmed in clinical studies that have shown that variceal hemorrhage does not occur when the HVPG is reduced to values under the threshold of 12 mm Hg[8,9] and that the risk for bleeding decreases significantly with the reduction of HVPG to more than 20% from baseline.[10]

Gastroesophageal varices are present in approximately 50% of patients with cirrhosis. Their presence correlates with the severity of liver disease; while only 40% of patients with Child's A disease have varices, they are present in 85% of Child's C disease patients.[11] Patients without varices develop them at a rate of 8% per year, and patients with small varices develop large varices at the same rate.[12,13]

Variceal hemorrhage occurs at a yearly rate of 5% to 15%, and the most important predictor of hemorrhage is the size of varices. A number of factors are used to predict variceal hemorrhage in patients with cirrhosis. These include physical, clinical, endoscopic, and hemodynamic factors (**Box 2**). An Italian group analyzed the endoscopic and clinical features that predicted the likelihood of bleeding prospectively.[1] Variceal size, presence of red wales, and Child-Pugh class were found to be predictive of variceal bleeding risk. The index defined by the study (Northern Italian Endoscopy Club [NIEC] index) has been prospectively validated and can be easily applied to research and clinical practice (**Table 1**).[1] This classification has, however, come under criticism because independent studies[14,15] have not confirmed the highly predictive values noted in the original study.[1]

DIAGNOSIS

A screening esophagogastroduodenoscopy (EGD) for the diagnosis of esophageal and gastric varices is recommended when the diagnosis of cirrhosis is made.[16] The NIEC has classified esophageal varices as F1, F2, and F3 (corresponding to small, medium, and large [> 5 mm]) with or without red signs (red wale marks, cherry-red

---

Box 2
Predictors of variceal hemorrhage

A. Physical

Elastic properties of the vessel

Intravariceal/intraluminal pressure

Variceal wall tension ($T = P \times R/W$)

B. Clinical

Continued alcohol use

Poor liver function (advanced Child's class)

Presence of ascites

C. Endoscopic

Large varices

Red signs (red wale markings)

D. Hemodynamic

HVPG >12 mm Hg

Table 1 Calculation of NIEC index[a]	
Variable	Points to Add
Child's class	
A	6.5
B	13.0
C	19.5
Size of varices	
Small	8.7
Medium	13.0
Large	17.4
Red wale markings	
Absent	3.2
Mild	6.4
Moderate	9.6
Severe	12.8

[a] NIEC index is computed by adding the 3 variables shown.
From The North Italian Endoscopic Club for the Study and Treatment of Esophageal Varices. Prediction of the first variceal hemorrhage in patients with cirrhosis of the liver and esophageal varices: a prospective multicenter study. N Engl J Med 1988;319:988; with permission.

spots or hematocystic spots). The frequency of surveillance endoscopies with no or small varices depends on their natural history. In patients with compensated cirrhosis who have no varices on screening endoscopy, the EGD should be repeated in 2 to 3 years. In those with small varices, the EGD should be repeated in 1 to 2 years and in the presence of decompensated cirrhosis, annually.[17] Endoscopic ultrasound has also been used to study varices and to identify increased risk for bleeding,[18] although it is unclear if this modality is superior to standard EGD. Esophageal capsule endoscopy is a promising technique, still evolving, which may provide an accurate, less invasive alternative to EGD.[19]

Gastric varices are classified by location according to the schema proposed by Sarin. Varices in direct continuity with the esophagus along the lesser and greater curvatures of the stomach are termed gastroesophageal varices (GOV) types 1 and 2, respectively. Isolated gastric varices (IGV) are a less common phenomenon and may be termed IGV1 when they occur in the fundus (often caused by splenic vein thrombosis or spontaneous splenorenal collaterals) or IGV2 (occurring in the gastric body, antrum, or duodenal bulb).[20]

Portal hypertensive gastropathy (PHG), the term used to describe the endoscopic appearance of gastric mucosa with a characteristic mosaic-like pattern with or without red spots, is a common finding in patients with portal hypertension.[21] The elementary lesions of PHG have been classified according to the NIEC classification.[22] A recent consensus statement of the Baveno III meeting on portal hypertension proposed a grading classification of PHG based on severity as "mild" or "severe."[17] Although the pathogenesis of PHG has not been clearly defined, a very close relationship exists between portal hypertension and the development of PHG. Although gastric antral vascular ectasia (GAVE) is a separate entity with a distinctly different management, the lesion of GAVE may mimic that of severe PHG, and a gastric biopsy may be required to differentiate them (as GAVE has a number of pathologic hallmarks).[21] Acute bleeding from PHG is often mild and self-limiting. Currently, the only treatment that could be recommended for prophylaxis of bleeding from PHG is nonselective β-blockers.[23]

PREPRIMARY PROPHYLAXIS

It is well established that varices do not develop until the HVPG exceeds 12 mm Hg. In animal models, the use of nonselective β-blockers has been shown to decrease the risk for the development of varices.[24] A large multicenter, placebo-controlled, double-blinded trial failed to show benefit of nonselective β-blockers (timolol) in the prevention of varices.[12] Thus, β-blockers are currently not recommended for preprimary prophylaxis.

PRIMARY PROPHYLAXIS

Therapy for primary prophylaxis against variceal bleeding has evolved considerably over the past decade.

Pharmacologic Therapy

The general objective of pharmacologic therapy for variceal bleeding is to reduce portal pressure and, consequently, intravariceal pressure.

The nonselective β-blockers have been the most widely studied medications in randomized controlled trials (RCTs) evaluating the efficacy of primary prophylaxis in patients with portal hypertension.[25] This class of medications reduces portal pressure by causing β-blockade, which allows unopposed α-adrenergic activity, thereby producing mesenteric arteriolar constriction that reduces portal venous flow (**Table 2**). At high doses, β-blockers also decrease blood pressure and cardiac output, further decreasing portal venous inflow and pressure. The 3 nonselective β-adrenergic blockers that have been used in clinical trials are nadolol, propranolol, and timolol. In the absence of determination of the HVPG, the dose of β-blockers is titrated on the basis of clinical measurements by incremental increases in dose to reach an end point of a resting heart rate of 55 beats per minute, a reduction of 25% from the baseline rate, or the development of side effects. In addition to their side effects, an important problem with β-blockers is their variable effect on portal pressure and the consequent difficulty in predicting a clinical response. Carvedilol, a nonselective β-blocker with intrinsic α1-adrenergic activity, has been shown to produce a greater decrease in portal pressure than propranolol, an effect probably related to an associated decrease in hepatic and portocollateral resistance. However, its use is clinically limited by its systemic hypotensive effects.[26]

Table 2
Effect on portal flow, resistance, and pressure with different therapies for varices/variceal hemorrhage

Treatment	Portal Flow	Portal Resistance	Portal Pressure
Vasoconstrictors (β-blockers)	↓↓	↑	↓
Venodilators (nitrates)	↓	↓	↓
Endoscopic therapy (band ligation/ sclerotherapy)	—	—	—
TIPS/shunt therapy	↑	↓↓↓	↓↓↓

From Garcia-Tsao G, Sanyal AJ, Grace ND, et al. Prevention and management of gastroesophageal varices and variceal hemorrhage in cirrhosis. Hepatology 2007;46(3):922–38; with permission.

A meta-analysis of trials evaluating nonselective β-blockers as primary prophylaxis analyzed the results of 3 trials that included patients with small varices.[27] The incidence of first variceal hemorrhage was 7% for 2 years and this was reduced to 2% with β-blockers (not statistically significant). Thus, the long-term benefit of β-blockers in this patient population has not been established.

A meta-analysis of 11 trials that included 1,189 patients evaluating nonselective β-blockers (ie, propranolol and nadolol) versus no active treatment or placebo in the prevention of first variceal hemorrhage showed that in patients with medium-sized or large varices, β-blockers reduce the risk for bleeding from 25% to 15% (relative risk reduction of 40%; number needed to treat [NNT]:10).[27] Mortality is also lesser in the β-blocker group[28] and β-blockers have been shown to be the only cost-effective form of prophylactic therapy.[29]

The use of β-blockers is limited by the small number of patients who have a hemodynamic response ($\sim$20%–30%), intolerance to therapy ($\sim$10%–20%) and rebound portal hypertension if stopped suddenly. Combination therapy with β-blockers and nitrates cannot be recommended because of the discrepant results of clinical trials.[30,31]

Endoscopic Therapy

Over the past 2 decades endoscopic therapy has assumed an increasingly prominent role in the treatment of esophageal varices. Both endoscopic sclerotherapy (ES) and endoscopic variceal ligation (EVL) have been shown to effectively eradicate varices. As primary prophylaxis, endoscopic therapy offers several distinct advantages over pharmacologic therapy. The duration of therapy is limited only to the time required for variceal obliteration (which improves compliance), and the need to measure hemodynamic parameters to assess response is obviated.

ES was first reported in 1939.[32] This method involves visualization of the varix during endoscopy, followed by injection of a sclerosing agent into the varix or into the adjacent tissue. Variceal obliteration is usually achieved after 3 to 6 sclerotherapy sessions at frequent intervals. Complications associated with ES include retrosternal pain, esophageal ulcers, esophageal stricture, and full-thickness necrosis resulting in perforation (exceptionally rare). The use of ES for the primary prophylaxis of variceal hemorrhage has been compared with no treatment in 22 RCTs. While early studies showed promising results, later studies showed no benefit,[33,34] and a Veterans Affairs (VA) prospective, randomized, cooperative trial was terminated prematurely because of an increased mortality rate in the ES group.[35] Based on these available data, ES is not recommended for primary prophylaxis.

EVL was first reported in 1989.[36] The technique involves the placement of rubber bands around a portion of the varix containing esophageal mucosa. The varix is sucked into a hollow, clear plastic cylinder attached to the tip of the endoscope. Once suctioned into the sheath, a trigger device allows deployment of the band around the varix. The blood flow is completely interrupted, producing ischemic necrosis of the mucosa and submucosa. Later granulation takes place with sloughing of the rubber rings and necrotic tissue, leaving shallow mucosal ulcerations that heal in 14 to 21 days. Initially, only a single band could be applied during esophageal intubation, leading to the need for an overtube. Subsequently, devices have been developed that allow for the application of as many as 10 bands during a single intubation. Application of the bands is started at the gastroesophageal junction and progresses cephalad in a helical fashion. EVL sessions are repeated at approximately 2-week intervals until varices are obliterated, usually requiring 2 to 4 ligation sessions. Complications are less frequent than with ES.

A recently published meta-analysis has examined the efficacy of band ligation in the primary prevention of variceal bleeding.[37] EVL reduces the risk for bleeding and improves survival compared with no treatment.[38] Meta-analysis of trials of EVL versus β-blockers shows that EVL reduces the risk for bleeding from 23% to 14% with a NNT of 11.[39] However, the survival was similar to that with β-blockers.

Although β-blockers remain the usual first-line therapy for primary prophylaxis, EVL is an acceptable alternative for patients at high-risk for variceal bleeding who have an intolerance of or contraindications to medical therapy.[16,40]

MANAGEMENT OF ACUTE VARICEAL HEMORRHAGE
General Measures

The initial resuscitative measures offer the earliest opportunity to influence the outcome of an episode of acute variceal bleeding (**Fig. 1** for a management algorithm). Many of the physiologic responses to hemorrhage may be impaired in patients with portal hypertension. A patient with suspected bleeding varices should be managed in an intensive care unit with appropriate expertise available in the medical and nursing staff. Initial resuscitation should follow the classic airway, breathing, circulation scheme and is aimed at restoring an appropriate delivery of oxygen to the tissues.

Airway protection should be provided, especially in encephalopathic patients, since the patient is at risk for bronchial aspiration of gastric contents and blood. Endotracheal intubation may be required electively or more urgently before endoscopic procedures. Blood volume replacement should be initiated as soon as possible with plasma expanders, aiming at maintaining a systolic blood pressure of approximately 100 mmHg. Avoiding prolonged hypotension is particularly important to prevent infection and renal failure, which are associated with increased risk for rebleeding and death.[41] Packed red cells are transfused conservatively to keep the target hemoglobin after transfusion around 9 gm/dL (hematocrit 25%–30%), as overtransfusion exacerbates portal hypertension and increases the risk for rebleeding.[42] Fresh frozen plasma and platelets, although frequently used, do not reliably correct coagulopathy and can induce volume overload.[43] A multicenter placebo-controlled trial of recombinant factor VIIa (rFVIIa) in patients with cirrhosis and gastrointestinal hemorrhage failed to show a beneficial effect versus standard therapy.[44] Although a post hoc analysis of a subpopulation of Child's B and C patients with cirrhosis indicated that administration of rFVIIa significantly decreased the proportion of patients with failure to control variceal bleeding, confirmatory studies are needed before this expensive therapy can be recommended in patients with coagulopathy and variceal bleeding.[16]

Cirrhosis is frequently associated with defects in both humoral and cellular host defense, hence increasing the risk for infection. This is particularly common at the time of or in the immediate days following a gastrointestinal hemorrhage.[45] The most frequent infections are spontaneous bacterial peritonitis (50%), urinary tract infections (25%), and pneumonia (25%). The use of prophylactic antibiotics in patients with acute variceal bleeding has been shown to reduce both the risk for rebleeding[46] and mortality.[47] Therefore, short-term antibiotic prophylaxis should be considered standard practice. Quinolones are frequently used because of their ease of administration and low cost.[48] In high-risk patients, intravenous ceftriaxone has been shown to be superior to oral norfloxacin.[49]

Specific Therapy for Control of Bleeding

The measures used to manage an episode of variceal bleeding may be classified into those that have an effect on variceal bleeding only during the period in which they are

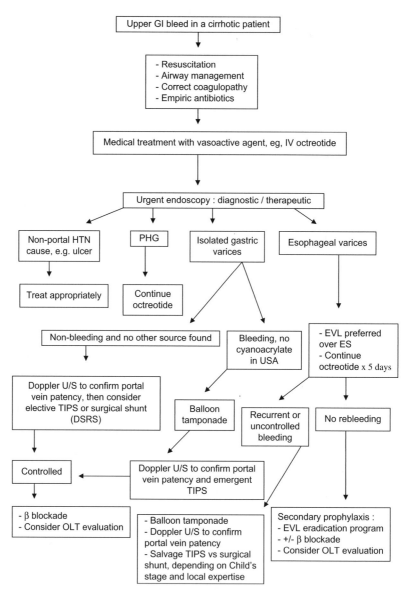

Fig. 1. Management algorithm for presumed acute variceal bleeding.

applied, and those that reduce the risk for early (hours to days) or long-term (weeks to months) recurrent hemorrhage. The clinical implications of this distinction are important, as those measures which have only short-term benefit should be followed by a more definitive procedure to prevent the high incidence of early rebleeding.

Measures Effective Only During the Period Applied

Pharmacologic therapy

Vasoactive drugs act to reduce variceal pressure by decreasing variceal blood flow. The selection of the drug depends on the local resources. Pharmacotherapy has the advantage of being initiated early, as soon as the diagnosis of variceal hemorrhage is suspected, even before diagnostic EGD.

Vasopressin and related compounds Vasopressin is the most potent splanchnic vasoconstrictor. It reduces blood flow to all splanchnic organs, thereby decreasing portal venous inflow and portal pressure. The clinical usefulness of the drug is limited by its multiple side effects related to its potent vasoconstrictor properties. These include hypertension, myocardial ischemia (and failure), arrhythmias, ischemic abdominal pain, and limb gangrene. Such complications are responsible for drug withdrawal in 25% of cases. Vasopressin has now mostly been abandoned as monotherapy. The concept of combining vasopressin and a vasodilator was developed with the aim of reducing the elevated rate of cardiovascular complications. Nitroglycerin was shown to reverse the systemic hemodynamic effects of vasopressin while the fall in portal pressure was maintained or enhanced.[50] This is because of the mainly venous dilator effect of nitroglycerin, which results in a reduction of portocollateral resistance and portal pressure. Three RCTs have been performed comparing the effects of vasopressin alone with vasopressin combined with nitroglycerin. All 3 showed that the combination had beneficial effects either for controlling bleeding and/or reducing vasopressin-associated complications. Nevertheless the observed benefits did not result in improvement in mortality.[51–53] There is ample justification to suggest that vasopressin should always be used in combination with nitroglycerin. Because of its short half-life, vasopressin is administered as a continuous intravenous infusion (0.4–0.8 U/min) while nitroglycerin should be administered by simultaneous intravenous infusion or transdermally.

Terlipressin (Glypressin) is a synthetic vasopressin analog with a longer biologic half-life and possessing far fewer side effects. The longer half-life allows the intravenous administration of the drug in bolus dosing, 2 mg every 4 to 6 hours until 24 hours free from bleeding is achieved. The clinical efficacy of terlipressin versus placebo has been assessed in 7 RCTs, and a meta-analysis showed that terlipressin significantly reduced failure to control bleeding and mortality.[54] It is important to note that terlipressin is the only pharmacologic agent that has been shown to reduce mortality (a 34% reduction). It is, however, currently not available in the United States.

Somatostatin and related analogs Somatostatin, a naturally occurring peptide, was introduced for the treatment of variceal hemorrhage because of its capacity to decrease portal pressure without the adverse effects of vasopressin on the systemic circulation. Its effects are probably achieved by 2 means: first, by inhibiting the release of splanchnic vasodilators such as glucagon, and second, by a direct splanchnic vasoconstrictor effect. The treatment regimen consists of bolus injections of 250 µg, followed by 250 µg/h administered as a continuous intravenous infusion. If successful, therapy is maintained for days. Major side effects are rare, and minor side effects, such as nausea, vomiting, and hyperglycemia, occur in about 30%.[55] Several RCTs have shown its efficacy in the control of bleeding; however, somatostatin did not reduce mortality.[27]

Octreotide and vapreotide are cyclic synthetic somatostatin analogs with longer half-lives than native somatostatin. Of these, only octreotide is available in the United States. The most commonly recommended schedule is as a 50 µg IV bolus, followed by a continuous intravenous infusion at 50 µg/h for 5 days. The efficacy of octreotide as a single therapy for variceal bleeding is controversial, which may be because of the rapid development of tachyphylaxis.[56] However, octreotide appears to be useful as an adjunct to endoscopic therapy (ES or EVL),[57] and a combination of EVL and octreotide (in the United States) as multimodality treatment is the preferred first-line approach to achieve hemostasis.

Balloon tamponade

The use of a Sengstaken-Blakemore or Minnesota tube can be a life-saving maneuver if medical and endoscopic measures fail to arrest the hemorrhage. Balloon tamponade of bleeding gastric or esophageal varices has been in widespread use since its introduction more than 40 years ago. Control of variceal bleeding has been reported in up to 90% of cases,[58] but rebleeding occurs in up to 50% when the balloons are deflated. The use of these tubes should be limited to experienced personnel, and endotracheal intubation of these patients is encouraged to decrease the risk for pulmonary aspiration injury. Complications occur in up to 30% of cases. The most frequently observed complication of this procedure is the occurrence of aspiration pneumonia, and this is best avoided by the use of elective endotracheal intubation in patients with grade III and IV encephalopathy. Other complications include airway obstruction (by a displaced esophageal balloon), esophageal necrosis/perforation, and mucosal ulceration (which may be a cause for rebleeding). Balloon tamponade is usually reserved as a life-saving, temporizing measure when a patient is exsanguinating. This may allow subsequent transjugular intrahepatic portosystemic shunts (TIPS) or surgical shunting. No other treatment can provide such immediate hemostasis in these circumstances— but at a high risk for complication to the patient.

Measures with Additional Effect on Rebleeding

Endoscopic therapy

The cornerstone of current management of variceal bleeding is endoscopy with active treatment. Endoscopic therapy has revolutionized the care of patients with cirrhosis and acute variceal hemorrhage and is capable of stopping bleeding in nearly 90% of patients. Accurate diagnosis is important, as other causes of gastrointestinal bleeding should be considered despite the presence of stigmata of portal hypertension.

ES, the technique which was previously described, arrests hemorrhage in 80% to 90% of patients[27] and decreases the risk for early rebleeding, although an improvement in patient survival has never been shown. ES has been shown to be superior to both vasopressin and balloon tamponade.[27] No sclerosing agent has been definitively shown to be superior to another.[59] There is a 10% to 30% complication rate (the major drawback of this modality) and a 0.5% to 2% mortality rate associated with ES. The complications have been described previously.

EVL, previously described, is a relatively newer therapeutic modality and has largely replaced ES as the preferred form of endoscopic management, as it is easier to perform and incurs a lesser complication rate. A recent meta-analysis of 10 RCTs comparing EVL with ES found an almost significant benefit of EVL in the initial control of bleeding with fewer complications.[60] Therefore, by consensus, EVL is the preferred form of endoscopic therapy.[16,40]

GOV1 gastric varices may be treated like esophageal varices; however, GOV2 gastric varices are located deeper in the submucosa than esophageal varices, and ES and EVL are usually ineffective in controlling them when bleeding acutely. Tissue adhesives (N-butyl-2-cyanoacrylate and isobutyl-2-cyanoacrylate) have been shown to be effective for bleeding gastric varices,[61] but no data are available from a randomized trial. In Europe and Canada these agents have been used with some success for treating gastric varices; however, drawbacks include the potential for systemic effects (such as embolic complications) and the risk for significant damage to the endoscope from exposure to tissue adhesives. For these reasons, cyanoacrylate glue is currently unavailable for use in the United States. The use of bovine fibrin or fibrin glue has also been reported by numerous centers.[62] Endoscopic ligation with a detachable mini-snare has, in addition, been described as a therapeutic option for bleeding gastric varices.[63] In the absence of these agents, TIPS should be considered first-line therapy for bleeding gastric varices.

Rescue therapies

Despite urgent endoscopic and/or pharmacologic therapy, variceal bleeding cannot be controlled or recurs in about 10% to 20% of patients. An elevated HVPG of more than 20 mmHg has been shown to be predictive of treatment failure.[64] Shunt therapy, either as shunt surgery (in Child's A patients) or TIPS, has clinical efficacy as salvage therapy. TIPS is a radiologic procedure by which a tract is created between the hepatic vein and portal vein and kept open by deployment of a coated stent, and it produces hemostasis in over 90% of cases.[65,66] TIPS-related complications include procedural complications (in about 10%)[67] and later TIPS dysfunction or stenosis. The latter occurs less frequently in the era of polytetrafluoroethylene(PTFE)-covered stents. The most frequent complication encountered is that of worsening encephalopathy, which occurs in about 25% of patients following TIPS placement.[68] The symptoms are usually mild and easily controlled with lactulose therapy and dietary protein restriction.

The surgical options currently used to treat variceal bleeding are either shunt or non-shunt procedures. The shunt operations are either total, including portacaval shunt, narrow-diameter portacaval shunt, mesocaval shunt, and central splenorenal shunt, or selective, including the distal splenorenal shunt (DSRS) and coronary caval shunt. The nonshunt operations are primarily gastroesophageal devascularization or disconnection procedures.[69] The DSRS is the principal selective shunt, and it controls variceal bleeding by selectively decompressing gastroesophageal varices (through the short gastric veins, the spleen and the splenic vein to the left renal vein) while simultaneously maintaining portal hypertension and portal flow to the cirrhotic liver.[70] In patients with nonalcoholic liver disease, portal perfusion is maintained in 85% of patients, allowing a lower rate of encephalopathy (<10%) compared with total shunts.[71] DSRS is associated with a low risk for operative morbidity, lesser shunt dysfunction rate, and good long-term patient survival.[72]

A large multicenter trial of TIPS versus DSRS (the DIVERT study) showed similar rates of rebleeding, encephalopathy, and mortality in patients with Child's A and B cirrhosis who had failed pharmacologic/endoscopic therapy, with a higher rate of shunt dysfunction in the TIPS group.[73] Because both procedures have equivalent outcomes, the choice is dependent on available local expertise.

SECONDARY PROPHYLAXIS

The natural history following the onset of variceal hemorrhage may be divided into 2 phases:[2] an acute phase, which lasts approximately 6 weeks, and the long-term course. The former is characterized by a high probability of recurrent hemorrhage after a short period of hemostasis. The risk for such early rebleeding is greatest in the first 48 hours after admission. The median rebleeding rate in untreated individuals is around 60% within 1 to 2 years of the index hemorrhage, with a mortality of 33%.[27,74] The prevention of recurrent variceal hemorrhage remains the cornerstone of management of such patients, and "secondary prophylaxis" should be instituted after the initial episode.

Pharmacologic Therapy

All patients who are deemed compliant and have no contraindications should be considered for pharmacologic therapy. Nonselective β-blockers reduce the relative risk for bleeding by 33% with an NNT of 4.76.[27] In a study by Poynard et al, evaluating those factors associated with rebleeding in patients receiving propranolol for secondary prophylaxis, presence of hepatocellular carcinoma, poor patient compliance, lack of a persistent decrease in pulse, and continued alcohol use were the factors identified.[75] The addition of isosorbide mononitrate (ISMN) to β-blockers appears to enhance the protective effect of β-blockers alone for the prevention of recurrent variceal bleeding but offers no survival advantage and reduces the tolerability of therapy.[76]

Endoscopic and Combination Endoscopic/Pharmacologic Therapy

EVL reduces the relative risk (vs sclerotherapy) for rebleeding by 37% and the absolute risk by 13% (NNT of 8).[77] Combination therapy of EVL and β-blockers is superior to EVL alone.[78] Combination of β-blockers (± nitrates) and ES has now been supplanted by EVL with β-blockers.

Other Salvage Therapies

TIPS or shunt surgery should be considered in patients with Child's A or B who experience recurrent variceal hemorrhage despite combination pharmacologic and endoscopic therapy.[79] Patients who are otherwise transplant candidates should be referred to a transplant center for evaluation. The goal of long-term treatment after an acute variceal bleed is prevention of rebleeding, hepatic decompensation, and death. Orthotopic liver transplantation is the only treatment that reliably achieves all 3 objectives. Thus, patients with Child's B or C cirrhosis should be evaluated for transplantation.

SUMMARY

Gastroesophageal variceal hemorrhage is a common and devastating complication of portal hypertension and is a leading cause of death in patients with cirrhosis. Many advances in the management of portal hypertension have occurred in the last 10 years. Although the role of EVL in primary prophylaxis is not established, effective therapy in the form of nonselective β-blockers is well accepted. The treatment of acute variceal bleeding is aimed at volume resuscitation, correction of coagulopathy, ensuring hemostasis with pharmacologic agents (such as somatostatin and its analogs), and endoscopic therapy (EVL being preferred over ES). TIPS and surgery are reserved as salvage therapy for endoscopic failures. Survivors of a variceal hemorrhage should be evaluated for liver transplantation. Because there is a high risk for recurrence after the initial hemorrhage, preventive strategies (including a variety of pharmacologic, endoscopic, and interventional approaches) are required and should be tailored to the patient's clinical condition, surgical risk, and prognosis.

REFERENCES

1. North Italian Endoscopic Club for the Study and Treatment of Esophageal Varices. Prediction of first variceal hemorrhage with cirrhosis of the liver and esophageal varices. N Engl J Med 1988;319:983–9.
2. Graham D, Smith J. The course of patients after variceal hemorrhage. Gastroenterology 1981;80:800–9.
3. Garcia N, Sanyal AJ. Portal hypertension. Clin Liver Dis 2001;5:509–40.

4. Groszmann RJ, Glickman M, Blei AT, et al. Wedged and free hepatic venous pressure measured with a balloon catheter. Gastroenterology 1979;76:253–8.
5. Garcia-Tsao G, Groszmann RJ, Fisher RL, et al. Portal pressure, presence of gastroesophageal varices and variceal bleeding. Hepatology 1985;5:419–24.
6. Viallet A, Marleau D, Huet M, et al. Hemodynamic evaluation of patients with intrahepatic portal hypertension: relationship between bleeding varices and the portohepatic gradient. Gastroenterology 1975;69:1297–300.
7. Polio J, Groszmann RJ. Hemodynamic factors involved in the development and rupture of esophageal varices: a pathophysiologic approach to treatment. Semin Liver Dis 1986;6:318–31.
8. Casado M, Bosch J, Garcia-Pagan JC, et al. Clinical events after transjugular intrahepatic portosystemic shunt: correlation with hemodynamic findings. Gastroenterology 1998;114:1296–303.
9. Groszmann RJ, Bosch J, Grace ND, et al. Hemodynamic events in a prospective randomized trial of propranolol vs placebo in the prevention of the first variceal hemorrhage. Gastroenterology 1990;99:1401–7.
10. Feu F, Garcia-Pagan JC, Bosch J, et al. Relationship between portal pressure response to pharmacotherapy and risk of recurrent variceal hemorrhage in patients with cirrhosis. Lancet 1995;346:1056–9.
11. Cales P, Zabotto B, Meskens C, et al. Gastroesophageal endoscopic features in cirrhosis: observer variability, interassociations, and relationship to hepatic dysfunction. Gastroenterology 1990;98:156–62.
12. Groszmann RJ, Garcia-Tsao G, Bosch J, et al. Beta blockers to prevent gastroesophageal varices in patients with cirrhosis. N Engl J Med 2005;353:2254–61.
13. Merli M, Nicolini G, Angeloni S, et al. Incidence and natural history of small esophageal varices in cirrhotic patients. J Hepatol 2003;38:266–72.
14. Colombo E, Casiraghi MA, Minoli G, et al. First bleeding episode from esophageal varices in cirrhotic patients: a prospective study of endoscopic predictive factors. Ital J Gastroenterol 1995;27:345–8.
15. Rigo GP, Merighi A, Chahin NJ, et al. A prospective study of the ability of three endoscopic classifications to predict hemorrhage from esophageal varices. Gastrointest Endosc 1992;38:425–9.
16. Garcia-Tsao G, Sanyal AJ, Grace ND, et al. Prevention and management of gastroesophageal varices and variceal hemorrahge in cirrhosis. Hepatology 2007;46(3):922–38.
17. de Franchis R. Updating consensus in portal hypertension: report of the Baveno III consensus workshop on definitions, methodology and therapeutic strategies in portal hypertension. J Hepatol 2000;33:846–52.
18. Rigau J, Bosch J, Bordas JM, et al. Endoscopic measurement of variceal pressure in cirrhosis: correlation with portal pressure and variceal hemorrhage. Gastroenterology 1989;96:873–80.
19. Eisen GM, Eliakim R, Zaman A. The accuracy of Pillcam ESO capsule endoscopy versus conventional upper endoscopy for the diagnosis of esophageal varices: a prospective three-center pilot study. Endoscopy 2006;38:31–5.
20. Sarin SK, Lahoti D, Saxena SP, et al. Prevalence, classification and natural history of gastric varices: a long-term follow-up study in 568 portal hypertension patients. Hepatology 1992;16:1343–9.
21. Thuluvath PJ, Yoo HY. Portal hypertensive gastropathy. Am J Gastroenterol 2002; 97:2973–8.
22. Carpinelli L, Primignani M, Preatoni P, et al. Portal hypertensive gastropathy: reproducibility of a classification, prevalence of elementary lesions, sensitivity

and specificity in the diagnosis of cirrhosis of the liver. A NIEC multicenter study. Ital J Gastroenterol Hepatol 1997;29:533–40.

23. Perez-Ayuso RM, Pique JM, Bosch J, et al. Propranolol in the prevention of recurrent bleeding from severe portal hypertensive gastropathy in cirrhosis. Lancet 1991;337:1431–4.

24. Sarin SK, Groszmann RJ, Mosca PG, et al. Propranolol ameliorates the development of portal-systemic shunting in a chronic murine schistosomiasis model of portal hypertension. J Clin Invest 1991;87:1032–6.

25. Shahi HM, Sarin SK. Prevention of first variceal bleed: an appraisal of current therapies. Am J Gastroenterol 1998;93:2348–58.

26. Banares R, Moitinho E, Matilla A, et al. Randomized comparison of long-term carvedilol and propranolol administration in the treatment of portal hypertension in cirrhosis. Hepatology 2002;36:1367–73.

27. D'Amico G, Pagliaro L, Bosch J. Pharmacological treatment of portal hypertension: an evidence-based approach. Semin Liver Dis 1999;19:475–505.

28. Chen W, Nikolova D, Frederiksen SL, et al. Beta-blockers reduce mortality in cirrhotic patients with esophageal varices who have never bled (Cochrane review). J Hepatol 2004;40(Suppl 1):67 [abstract].

29. Teran JC, Imperiale TF, Mullen KD, et al. Primary prophylaxis of variceal bleeding in cirrhosis: a cost-effectiveness analysis. Gastroenterology 1997; 112:473–82.

30. Garcia-Pagan JC, Morillas R, Banares R, et al. Propranolol plus placebo vs propranolol plus isosorbide-5-mononitrate in the prevention of a first variceal bleed: a double-blind RCT. Hepatology 2003;37:1260–6.

31. D'Amico G, Pasta L, Politi F, et al. Isosorbide mononitrate with nadolol compared to nadolol alone for prevention of first bleeding in cirrhosis. A double-blind placebo-controlled randomized trial. Gastroenterol Int 2002;15:40–50.

32. Crafoord C, Frenckner P. New surgical treatment of varicose veins of the esophagus. Acta Otolaryngol (Stockholm) 1939;27:422.

33. D'Amico G, Pagliaro L, Bosch J. The treatment of portal hypertension: a meta-analytic review. Hepatology 1995;22:332–54.

34. Pagliaro L, D'Amico G, Sorensen TIA, et al. Prevention of first bleeding in cirrhosis. A meta-analysis of RCT's of non-surgical treatment. Ann Intern Med 1997;117:59–60.

35. The VA. Cooperative Variceal Sclerotherapy Group. Prophylactic sclerotherapy for esophageal varices in men with alcoholic liver disease. A randomized, single-blind, multicenter clinical trial. N Engl J Med 1991;324:1779–84.

36. Stiegmann GV, Goff JS, Sun JH, et al. Technique and early clinical results of endoscopic variceal ligation (EVL). Surg Endosc 1989;3:73–8.

37. Imperiale TF, Chalasani N. A meta-analysis of endoscopic variceal ligation for primary prophylaxis of esophageal variceal bleeding. Hepatology 2001;33: 802–7.

38. Sarin SK, Lamba GS, Kumar M, et al. Comparison of endoscopic ligation and propranolol for the primary prevention of variceal bleeding. N Engl J Med 1999;340:988–93.

39. Khuroo MS, Khuroo NS, Farahat KL, et al. Meta-analysis: endoscopic variceal ligation for primary prophylaxis of esophageal variceal bleeding. Aliment Pharmacol Ther 2005;21:347–61.

40. de Franchis R. Evolving consensus in portal hypertension: report of the Baveno IV consensus workshop on methodology of diagnosis and therapy in portal hypertension. J Hepatol 2005;43:167–76.

41. Cardenas A, Gines P, Uriz J, et al. Renal failure after upper gastrointestinal bleeding in cirrhosis: incidence, clinical course, predictive factors and short-term prognosis. Hepatology 2001;34:671–6.
42. Kravetz D, Sikuler E, Groszmann RJ. Splanchnic and systemic hemodynamics in portal hypertensive rats during hemorrhage and blood volume resuscitation. Gastroenterology 1986;90:1232–40.
43. Youssef WI, Salazar F, Dasarathy S, et al. Role of fresh frozen plasma infusion in correction of coagulopathy of chronic liver disease: a dual phase study. Am J Gastroenterol 2003;98:1391–4.
44. Bosch J, Thabut D, Bendtsen F, et al. Recombinant factor VIIa for upper gastro-intestinal bleeding in patients with cirrhosis: a randomized, double-blind trial. Gastroenterology 2004;127:1123–30.
45. Bleicher G, Boulanger R, Squara P, et al. Frequency of infections in cirrhotic patients presenting with acute gastrointestinal hemorrhage. Br J Surg 1986;73:724–6.
46. Hou MC, Lin HC, Liu TT, et al. Antibiotic prophylaxis after endoscopic therapy prevents rebleeding in acute variceal hemorrhage: a randomized trial. Hepatology 2004;39:746–53.
47. Bernard B, Grange JD, Khac EN, et al. Antibiotic prophylaxis for the prevention of bacterial infections in cirrhotic patients with gastrointestinal bleeding: a meta-analysis. Hepatology 1999;29:1655–61.
48. Rimola A, Garcia-Tsao G, Navasa M, et al. Diagnosis, treatment and prophylaxis of spontaneous bacterial peritonitis: a consensus document. International Ascites Club. J Hepatol 2000;32:142–53.
49. Fernandez J, Ruiz-del-Arbol L, Gomez C, et al. Norfloxacin vs ceftriaxone in the prophylaxis of infections in patients with advanced cirrhosis and hemorrhage. Gastroenterology 2006;131:1049–56.
50. Groszmann R, Kravetz D, Bosch J, et al. Nitroglycerin improves hemodynamic response to vasopressin in portal hypertension. Hepatology 1982;2:757–62.
51. Gimson A, Westaby D, Hegarty J, et al. A randomized trial of vasopressin and vasopressin plus nitroglycerin in the control of acute variceal hemorrhage. Hepatology 1986;6:410–3.
52. Tsai Y, Lay K, Ng W, et al. Controlled trial of vasopressin plus nitroglycerin vs vasopressin alone in the treatment of bleeding esophageal varices. Hepatology 1986;6:406–9.
53. Bosch J, Groszmann R, Garcia-Pagan JC, et al. Association of transdermal nitro-glycerin to vasopressin infusion in the treatment of variceal hemorrhage: a placebo-controlled clinical trial. Hepatology 1989;10:962–8.
54. Ioannou GN, Doust J, Rockey DC. Systematic review: terlipressin in acute esoph-ageal variceal hemorrhage. Aliment Pharmacol Ther 2003;17:53–64.
55. Moitinho E, Planas R, Banares R, et al. Multicenter randomized controlled trial comparing different schedules of somatostatin in the treatment of acute variceal bleeding. J Hepatol 2001;35:712–8.
56. Escorsell A, Bandi JC, Andreu V, et al. Desensitization to the effects of intrave-nous octreotide in cirrhotic patients with portal hypertension. Gastroenterology 2001;120:161–9.
57. Banares R, Albillos A, Rincon D, et al. Endoscopic treatment versus endoscopic plus pharmacologic treatment for acute variceal bleeding: a meta-analysis. Hep-atology 2002;305:609–15.
58. Avgerinos A, Armonis A. Balloon tamponade technique and efficacy in variceal hemorrhage. Scand J Gastroenterol Suppl 1994;207:11–6.

59. Sarin SK, Kumar A. Sclerosants for variceal sclerotherapy; a critical appraisal. Am J Gastroenterol 1990;85:641–9.

60. Garcia-Pagan JC, Bosch J. Endoscopic band ligation in the treatment of portal hypertension. Nat Clin Pract Gastroenterol Hepatol 2005;2:526–35.

61. Huang YH, Yeh HZ, Chen GH, et al. Endoscopic treatment of bleeding gastric varices by N-butyl-2-cyanoacrylate (Histoacryl) injection; long-term efficacy and safety. Gastrointest Endosc 2000;52:160–7.

62. Zimmer T, Rucktaschel F, Stolzel U, et al. Endoscopic sclerotherapy with fibrin glue as compared with polidocanol to prevent early esophageal variceal rebleeding. J Hepatol 1998;28:292.

63. Cipoletta L, Bianco MA, Rotondano G, et al. Emergency endoscopic ligation of actively bleeding varices with a detachable snare. Gastrointest Endosc 1998; 47:400–3.

64. Moitinho E, Escorsell A, Bandi JC, et al. Prognostic value of early measurements of portal pressure in acute variceal bleeding. Gastroenterology 1999; 117:626–31.

65. Bureau C, Garcia-Pagan JC, Otal P, et al. Improved clinical outcome using PTFE-coated stents for TIPS: results of a randomized study. Gastroenterology 2004; 126:469–75.

66. Sanyal AJ, Freedman AM, Luketic VA, et al. Transjugular intrahepatic portosystemic shunts for patients with active variceal hemorrhage unresponsive to sclerotherapy. Gastroenterology 1996;111:138–46.

67. Freedman AM, Sanyal AJ, Tisnado J, et al. Complications of transjugular intrahepatic portosystemic shunt: a comprehensive review. Radiographics 1993;13: 1185–210.

68. Rössle M, Haag K, Ochs A, et al. The transjugular intrahepatic portosystemic stent-shunt procedure for variceal bleeding. N Engl J Med 1993;330: 165–71.

69. Iannitti DA, Henderson JM. The role of surgery in the treatment of portal hypertension. Clinics in Liver Disease 1997;1:99–114.

70. Warren WD, Zeppa R, Foman JS. Selective transplenic decompression of gastroesophageal varices by distal splenorenal shunt. Ann Surg 1967;166:437–55.

71. Conn HO, Resnick RH, Grace ND, et al. Distal splenorenal shunt vs. portalsystemic shunt; current status of a controlled trial. Hepatology 1981;1:151–60.

72. Millikan WJ, warren WD, Henderson JM, et al. The Emory prospective randomized trial: selective versus nonselective shunt to control variceal bleeding: ten year follow-up. Ann Surg 1985;201:712–22.

73. Henderson JM, Boyer TD, Kutner MH, et al. Distal spelorenal shunt versus transjugular intrahepatic portosystemic shunt for variceal bleeding: a randomized trial. Gastroenterology 2006;130:1643–51.

74. Bosch J, Garcia-Pagan JC. Prevention of variceal bleeding. Lancet 2003;361: 952–4.

75. Poynard T, Lebrec D, Hillon P, et al. Propranolol for prevention of recurrent gastrointestinal bleeding in patients with cirrhosis. A prospective study of factors associated with rebleeding. Hepatology 1987;7:447–51.

76. Gournay J, Masliah C, Martin T, et al. Isosorbide mononitrate and propranolol compared with propranolol alone for the prevention of variceal rebleeding. Hepatology 2000;31:1239–45.

77. Laine L, Cook D. Endoscopic ligation compared with sclerotherapy for treatment of esophageal variceal bleeding. A meta-analysis. Ann Intern Med 1995;123: 280–7.

78. Lo GH, Lai KH, Cheng JS, et al. Endscopic variceal ligation plus nadolol and sucralfate compared with ligation alone for the prevention of variceal rebleeding: a prospective, randomized trial. Hepatology 2000;32:461–5.

79. Luca A, D'Amico G, La Galla R, et al. TIPS for the prevention of recurrent bleeding in patients with cirrhosis: meta-analysis of randomized clinical trials. Radiology 1999;212:411–21.

Renal Failure in Patients with Cirrhosis

Lina Mackelaite, MD[a], Zygimantas C. Alsauskas, MD[b],
Karthik Ranganna, MD[a],*

KEYWORDS

- Renal failure • Cirrhosis • Hepatorenal syndrome
- Glomerular disease • Hepatitis B virus • Hepatitis C virus

Renal failure is a common occurrence in patients with cirrhosis. It is caused by a variety of factors, some specific to cirrhosis, and others affecting the general patient population. Renal failure in cirrhosis connotes a worse prognosis; mortality is especially high with hepatorenal syndrome (HRS). Patients with cirrhosis who develop renal failure pose unique diagnostic and therapeutic challenges.

ASSESSMENT OF RENAL FUNCTION IN PATIENTS WITH CIRRHOSIS

Clinical measures tend to overestimate renal function in patients with cirrhosis, including laboratory values (serum creatinine and blood urea nitrogen levels), creatinine clearance calculated from timed urine collection, estimated creatinine clearance (using the Cockcroft-Gault formula), and estimated glomerular filtration rate (GFR). As a result, renal failure is often underdiagnosed in cirrhosis. Predictive equations (Modification of Diet in Renal Disease [MDRD], Cockcroft-Gault) can only be used when renal function is stable (steady state) and should not be used in acute renal failure, when creatinine is rising.[1]

Creatinine is produced in patients with cirrhosis at half the normal rate.[2] Possible reasons are malnutrition, low muscle mass, and impaired synthesis of creatine in cirrhotic liver.[3] Lower serum creatinine values lead to overestimation of renal function by predictive equations. As renal function declines in cirrhosis, tubular secretion of creatinine increases, which can result in higher creatinine clearance calculated from timed urine collection compared with true GFR.[4]

In 13 patients with cirrhosis and mean creatinine values of 1.1 ± 0.1 mg/dL, mean GFR by inulin clearance was 32 ± 4 mL/min, indicating that "normal" creatinine is a poor predictor of normal renal function.[5] In the same group of patients, creatinine

[a] Division of Nephrology, Department of Medicine, Drexel University College of Medicine, 245 North 15th Street, Room 6144, Philadelphia, PA 19102, USA
[b] Division of Nephrology, Department of Medicine, Mount Sinai School of Medicine, One Gustave L. Levy Place, Box 1243, New York, NY 10029, USA
* Corresponding author.
E-mail address: karthik.ranganna@drexelmed.edu (K. Ranganna).

Med Clin N Am 93 (2009) 855–869
doi:10.1016/j.mcna.2009.03.003
0025-7125/09/$ – see front matter © 2009 Elsevier Inc. All rights reserved.

medical.theclinics.com

clearance calculated from timed urine collection overestimated GFR by 96%, and use of the Cockcroft-Gault formula overestimated GFR by 208%.

A study of 1447 patients with cirrhosis about to undergo liver transplantation compared Cockcroft-Gault formula and 4-, 5-, and 6-variable MDRD equations with GFR measured by ^{125}I-iothalamate clearance.[6] In the subgroup with renal dysfunction (GFR < 40 mL/min), mean GFR was 22.6 ± 11.1 mL/min. Mean estimated creatinine clearance (Cockcroft-Gault) was 46.1 ± 27.1 mL/min, and mean estimated GFR (by 6-variable MDRD equation) was 39.0 ± 26.2 mL/min, grossly overestimating ^{125}I-iothalamate GFR.

In some reports cystatin C–based estimates predict GFR somewhat better than creatinine-based equations in patients with cirrhosis.[7,8] Evidence is insufficient to recommend cystatin C over other methods; however, this measurement is not available for routine use in clinical practice.

Creatinine measurement can be affected by hyperbilirubinemia. A study measured serum creatinine in 158 patients using 4 different creatinine assays.[9] Interassay agreement was poor and Model for End-Stage Liver Disease(MELD) score variability was high, especially with high bilirubin concentrations (> 400 μmol/L). The kinetic Jaffe method, most commonly used in the United States, is susceptible to bilirubin interference, which can lead to falsely low serum creatinine values when bilirubin concentration is 10 mg/dL or higher.[10] To avoid this problem, the enzymatic method should be used to measure serum creatinine when the bilirubin level is very high.

RENAL FAILURE AS A PROGNOSTIC INDICATOR IN CIRRHOSIS

Renal failure in cirrhosis confers increased risk of death. A study of 231 patients was conducted to devise a prediction model for 3-month mortality after placement of a transjugular intrahepatic portosystemic shunt.[11] Multivariate analysis showed increased creatinine to be one of the factors (along with bilirubin and international normalized ratio) independently associated with higher mortality. A 100% rise in serum creatinine increased the risk of death 1.94-fold. Findings of this study led to the development of the MELD score, which was subsequently validated in a cohort of liver transplantation candidates[12] and was adopted by the United Network for Organ Sharing (UNOS)[13] to allocate donor livers based on severity of disease of the potential recipient. Thus, patients with higher creatinine or those requiring renal replacement therapy (RRT) have higher priority to receive liver allograft.

Development of HRS significantly shortens survival in patients with cirrhosis. A study of 105 patients with HRS assessed prognostic factors and outcome in patients with cirrhosis and HRS.[14] In a multivariate analysis, type of HRS (type 1 vs type 2) and MELD score were the only independent prognostic factors. All patients with type 1 HRS had MELD scores of 20 or greater, and their median survival was 1 month. Survival with type 2 HRS was dependent on MELD score: patients with MELD scores of 20 or greater survived for a median of 3 months; for those with MELD scores lower than 20, median survival was 11 months.

Development of renal failure before liver transplantation has a negative impact on posttransplant outcomes. In a large retrospective review of UNOS database for adults undergoing orthotopic liver transplantation (OLT), moderate to severe renal failure at the time of OLT was associated with significantly lower short-term and long-term graft and patient survival rates.[15]

CLASSIFICATION

Based on etiology, renal failure is divided into prerenal, renal, and postrenal categories. Renal failure is caused by a variety of factors, some specific to cirrhosis (eg, hepatorenal syndrome), and others affecting the general patient population. Common causes of renal failure in patients with cirrhosis are listed below.

PRERENAL

- Vomiting, diarrhea, nasogastric suction
- Excessive diuresis
- Hemorrhage
- Circulatory dysfunction following large-volume paracentesis (LVP)
- HRS
- Abdominal compartment syndrome
- Medications causing hemodynamic changes, for example, nonsteroidal antiin-flammatory drugs (NSAIDs), angiotensin converting enzyme (ACE) inhibitors

INTRINSIC RENAL

- Glomerulonephritis
- Membranoproliferative glomerulonephritis (MPGN), cryoglobulinemia (hepatitis C virus [HCV]–related)
- Membranous nephropathy (hepatitis B virus [HBV]–related)
- IgA nephropathy
- Interstitial nephritis
- Acute tubular necrosis (ATN):
- Toxic ATN, for example, due to aminoglycoside or radiocontrast exposure
- Ischemic ATN, for example, in the setting of septic or hemorrhagic shock

POSTRENAL

- Benign prostatic hyperplasia
- Neurogenic bladder
- Nephrolithiasis
- Papillary necrosis in alcoholic liver disease

An episode of acute renal failure may be reversible, but renal function may remain diminished over the long term, and patients develop chronic kidney disease.

A suggested diagnostic approach to renal failure in cirrhosis is provided in **Fig. 1**.

Prerenal Causes

Excessive diuresis, vomiting, diarrhea, poor oral intake, and gastrointestinal hemorrhage may lead to extracellular fluid volume depletion and renal failure. In cirrhosis and portal hypertension, effective arterial blood volume (EABV) may be decreased, leading to renal hypoperfusion and failure even in the presence of gross extracellular fluid overload.

Diuretic Use

Extracellular fluid overload develops in patients with cirrhosis and portal hypertension. Increased local production of vasodilatory substances, mostly nitric oxide,[16] induces splanchnic vasodilation.[17] Decreased systemic vascular resistance, arterial hypotension, and low EABV activate the renin-angiotensin-aldosterone system,[18] the

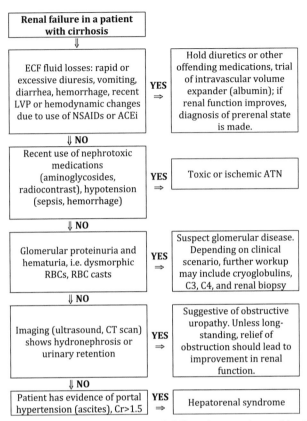

Fig. 1. Suggested diagnostic approach to renal failure in a patient with cirrhosis. ACE-I, angiotensin-converting enzyme inhibitor; ATN, acute tubular necrosis; Cr, creatinine; CT, computed tomography; ECF, extracellular fluid; GN, glomerulonephritis; LVP, large-volume paracentesis; NSAID, nonsteroidal antiinflammatory drug; RBC, red blood cell.

sympathetic nervous system,[19] and vasopressin,[20] leading to salt and water retention. Diuretics, usually a combination of furosemide and spironolactone, are the mainstay of therapy in volume-overloaded patients who are diuretic sensitive. Excessive or too rapid diuresis can lead to volume depletion, causing renal failure.

Patients with peripheral edema can tolerate more rapid diuresis than can patients with ascites alone. A study of 14 patients with cirrhosis treated with a combination of oral diuretics showed that edema fluid was preferentially mobilized. Patients with edema did not develop renal impairment or a decrease in plasma volume despite a mean negative fluid balance of 1.79 kg/d.[21] Patients with ascites, but no edema at enrollment, were prone to a decrease in plasma volume and to the development of reversible decline in renal function; mean negative balance was 1.27 kg/d. Extrapolating from the findings of this study, it is safe to achieve rapid diuresis ($\leq$ 2 L/d) when edema is present. In patients with ascites but no edema, negative balance should be kept at 750 mL/d or less.

Large-Volume Paracentesis

With progressive liver disease and increasing activity of endogenous neurohormonal systems, sodium avidity rises. Patients develop diuretic resistance, which is defined as the inability to achieve weight loss despite adherence to dietary salt restriction and maximum-dose diuretics.[22] In this setting, LVP is performed serially to alleviate discomfort and other problems associated with rapidly accumulating ascites. Sometimes LVP is performed in patients who are sensitive to diuretics to quickly relieve tense ascites. Following LVP, some patients develop a further decrease in intravascular volume, termed postparacentesis circulatory dysfunction, which may cause renal failure.

One study assessed the effect of volume expansion with albumin on postparacentesis circulatory dysfunction. One hundred five patients presenting with tense ascites were randomly assigned to undergo paracentesis (4–6 L/d until resolution of ascites) with or without albumin infusion (40 g) after each procedure.[23] Diuretic resistance was not a prerequisite to enter the study. Patients not receiving albumin developed a marked elevation in plasma renin activity and aldosterone level, indicating impairment in systemic hemodynamics. There was also a rise in blood urea nitrogen and a reduction in serum sodium with no albumin replacement. These changes were not seen in the group that received albumin infusions. No difference was found in survival between study groups. Until further evidence is available, intravenous albumin (10 g/L of fluid removed) may be considered for LVP but is not necessary for single paracentesis of less than 5 L.[24]

Hepatorenal Syndrome

Typically, HRS develops in advanced liver disease, when other complications of cirrhosis are already present, including ascites and hyponatremia.[25] Among patients with ascites, HRS develops in about 20% and 40% of the patients, at 1 and 5 years, respectively.[25]

Progressive liver disease causes a further decrease in systemic vascular resistance and activation of compensatory neurohormonal systems. Rising renal vasoconstriction and decreasing GFR culminates in HRS.[26] Relatively low and insufficient cardiac output may contribute to renal hypoperfusion in patients with cirrhosis who have HRS.[27] HRS is a functional disorder, without underlying structural kidney damage.

The most common trigger for the development of type-1 HRS is bacterial infection, mainly spontaneous bacterial peritonitis (SBP). According to a study of 252 SBP episodes in patients with cirrhosis, renal failure developed in 33% of the episodes, and had a progressive course in 14%.[28]

Diagnosis

Diagnosis of HRS is based on exclusion of other types of renal failure. Diagnostic criteria for HRS in cirrhosis were updated in a recent meeting of the International Ascites Club.[29]

- Cirrhosis with ascites
- Serum creatinine greater than 1.5 mg/dL
- No improvement in serum creatinine (to ≤1.5 mg/dL) after 2 days or more of diuretic withdrawal and volume expansion with albumin (1 g/kg/d, up to 100 g/d)
- Absence of shock
- No current or recent treatment with nephrotoxic drugs
- Absence of parenchymal kidney disease as indicated by proteinuria greater than 500 mg/d, microhematuria greater than 50 red blood cells per high-power field or abnormal renal ultrasonographic findings

The previous definition[22] was modified to allow the diagnosis of HRS when renal failure occurs in the setting of bacterial infection (eg, SBP) without shock, and hence facilitating earlier initiation of specific therapies for HRS without waiting for complete recovery from the infection. Creatinine clearance is no longer recommended for the diagnosis of HRS. The revised guidelines also recommend albumin over 0.9% saline as an intravascular volume expander. Minor diagnostic criteria, including oliguria and urine Na^+ values less than 10 mEq/L, were considered nonessential and therefore were eliminated.

Based on severity of renal impairment, HRS is arbitrarily divided into type 1 and type 2. Type 1 HRS is defined as rapidly progressive renal failure (doubling of the initial serum creatinine to a level > 2.5 mg/dL in less than 2 weeks). Type 2 HRS is characterized by moderate renal failure (creatinine 1.5–2.5 mg/dL) with a steady or slowly progressive course. It is often associated with refractory ascites.

Prevention

A study of 126 patients assessed the role of intravenous albumin in preventing HRS in the setting of SBP.[30] Patients were assigned to receive treatment either with cefotaxime alone or a combination of cefotaxime plus intravenous albumin infusion at a dose of 1.5 g/kg within 6 hours after randomization and repeat infusion at a dose of 1 g/kg on day 3. Progressive renal failure developed in 33% of patients in the cefotaxime group compared with 6% in the group receiving a combination of cefotaxime and albumin, despite rapid resolution of infection in both groups. In-hospital mortality was 29% in the cefotaxime group, as compared with 10% in the cefotaxime and albumin group. Addition of albumin significantly decreased plasma renin activity, compared with cefotaxime alone. In a subgroup of patients with bilirubin less than 4 mg/dL and creatinine less than 1 mg/dL, the risk of renal failure was very low, regardless of treatment strategy.

A randomized trial of 68 cirrhotic patients at high risk for HRS-1 and SBP compared daily norfloxacin to placebo for primary prophylaxis of SBP.[31] In addition to improved mortality and lower incidence of SBP, norfloxacin group was also found to have lower incidence of HRS at 1 year (28% vs 41%).

Treatment

General measures include withdrawal of diuretics and intravascular volume expansion with albumin to rule out prerenal component and discontinuation of nephrotoxic medications, including NSAIDs and aminoglycosides.

Numerous reports have been published on treating type-1 HRS patients with vasoconstrictors such as combined midodrine and octreotide,[32] terlipressin (a synthetic vasopressin analog),[33,34] and norepinephrine[35] to counteract splanchnic vasodilation, usually in combination with intravenous albumin. Although some of these reports demonstrate improvement in renal function with vasopressors, no clear survival benefit has been shown. Terlipressin is not currently available in the United States. It is a potential concern that vasopressor-induced improvement in creatinine may decrease MELD scores and delay liver transplantation in prospective recipients. Several sources[36,37] provide detailed summaries of previous studies of vasopressors in hepatorenal syndrome.

RRT is initiated for standard indications in patients with HRS (volume overload, electrolyte and acid-base disturbances).

The greatest chance to recover renal function and improve overall survival in patients with HRS is successful liver transplantation. In one retrospective review of HRS patients undergoing OLT, GFR increased from 19.9 ± 3.6 mL/min preoperatively to 32.5 ± 3.1 mL/min at 6 weeks and 45.9 ± 5.5 mL/min at 1 year following OLT.[38] Despite overall improvement in renal function in patients with HRS, 10% of HRS patients developed end-stage renal disease (ESRD) compared with 0.8% non-HRS patients posttransplant. Although the actuarial 1- and 2-year survival rates were 76.6% in HRS patients following OLT, they were still less when compared with patients without HRS (1- and 2-year survival rates of 87.2% and 82.1%, respectively).

Abdominal Compartment Syndrome

Abdominal compartment syndrome should be suspected in a patient with cirrhosis who has massive ascites and decreased urine output.[39] It is defined as sustained intra-abdominal pressure (IAP) of greater than 20 mm Hg, associated with new organ dysfunction.[40] Normal IAP in critically ill patients is 5 to 7 mm Hg. Renal impairment in patients with increased IAP occurs due to renal vein compression and arterial vaso-constriction, caused by activation of the sympathetic nervous system and the renin-angiotensin-aldosterone system.[41,42]

Severity of abdominal distention observed on physical examination does not aid in the diagnosis of abdominal compartment syndrome. In one study, IAP was assessed by physical examination in 128 postoperative patients in the intensive care unit.[43] Using transvesicular pressure measurement as a reference, the positive predictive value of physical examination to detect IAP greater than 18 mm Hg was 45.2%, and the negative predictive value was 88.6%. Thus, transvesicular pressure measurements are required to make the diagnosis. If abdominal compartment syndrome is suspected, LVP should be performed.

Intrinsic Renal Causes

Several glomerular diseases are associated with cirrhosis: IgA nephropathy, membranous nephropathy, and MPGN. HBV and HCV infections are most strongly linked to the development of membranous nephropathy and MPGN, respectively, and may occur in the absence of cirrhosis. Glomerular disease should be suspected in patients with hypertension, proteinuria, and glomerular hematuria (dysmorphic red blood cells and red blood cell casts), although in many cases glomerular changes are clinically silent.

IgA Nephropathy

Glomerular IgA deposits are frequently found in patients with cirrhosis, but clinically evident renal impairment is uncommon. In an autopsy series, predominant mesangial IgA deposits were found in 36% of 75 liver cirrhosis cases.[44] In another study, 30 patients with HCV cirrhosis underwent intraoperative renal biopsies during liver transplantation.[45] Seven of them had mesangial proliferation and IgA deposits, but only 2 had elevated serum creatinine levels with subnephrotic proteinuria, and only 1 patient had hematuria.

Pathogenesis of IgA nephropathy in cirrhosis remains poorly understood. Levels of circulating IgA are increased in the serum of patients with alcoholic liver disease compared with healthy controls.[46,47] In vitro studies of lymphocytes from patients with alcoholic cirrhosis show that IgA synthesis may be increased.[48] Circulating IgA levels are elevated in patients with cirrhosis, with increased fraction of polymeric IgA, decreased catabolism of polymeric IgA, and disproportionately higher rise in IgA2 compared with IgA1.[49] IgA2 is cleared mainly through the hepatic asialoglycopro-tein receptor, but only a small fraction of IgA1 is cleared through this pathway.[50] This may account for the higher proportion of circulating IgA2 compared with IgA1 in patients with cirrhosis. IgA1 is the predominant form in renal deposits.[51] IgA nephropathy in patients with cirrhosis can manifest as azotemia, hematuria, subnephrotic-range proteinuria, or overt nephrotic syndrome.[44,45,52–54]

No study has specifically addressed the treatment of IgA nephropathy in cirrhosis. In several case reports of cirrhosis, portal hypertension, and IgA nephropathy, proteinuria decreased after treatment with propranolol was started, possibly due to a favorable effect on portal hypertension.[52,53]

Glomerulonephritis in Patients with Cirrhosis and Hepatitis B or C Infection

Hepatitis C virus infection

Membranoproliferative glomerulonephritis with mixed essential cryoglobulinemia is most strongly, and likely causally, associated with HCV infection.[55,56] Membranous nephropathy,[57,58] focal segmental glomerulosclerosis,[59] and IgA nephropathy[45] have also been reported in the setting of HCV infection.

Glomerular changes were assessed in an autopsy series of 188 patients with HCV infection.[54] A total of 83.5% of cases had histologic evidence of liver cirrhosis. MPGN was found in 11.2% of all autopsy cases, membranous nephropathy in 2.7%, mesangioproliferative glomerulonephritis in 17.6%, mesangial expansion without proliferation in 23.4%, and normal glomeruli in the remaining 45.2% of cases. In the presence of cirrhosis, glomerulonephritis was found in 59.2% of the patients, in contrast to 32.3% among the patients without cirrhosis. Overall, 12.2% of patients had abnormal urinalysis findings (hematuria or proteinuria) within 1 year before death. Urinalysis findings were abnormal in 42% of patients with MPGN.

In another report, 30 patients had intraoperative kidney biopsy during liver transplantation for cirrhosis due to HCV infection.[45] Twenty-five of them had evidence of immune complex glomerulonephritis: 12 had MPGN type 1, 7 had IgA nephropathy, and 6 had mesangial glomerulonephritis. Fifteen of the 25 had normal urinalysis findings and no proteinuria by quantitative estimates.

Most patients with mixed essential cryoglobulinemia have evidence of HCV infection. HCV virions and immune complexes are found in high concentrations in the cryoprecipitates.[56] Glomerular HCV protein deposits were detected in 67% of cryoglobulinemic MPGN biopsy specimens, suggesting a possible causal role of HCV infection.[60]

Mixed essential cryoglobulinemia is a systemic vasculitis that can present with systemic symptoms, palpable purpura, and kidney disease. Patients have detectable cryoglobulins and rheumatoid factor as well as low C3 and C4 levels. Renal involvement manifests as hypertension, azotemia, proteinuria, and nephritic sediment.

The optimal strategy for the treatment of glomerular disease associated with HCV infection in cirrhosis is unknown. Most treatment reports have focused on patients without cirrhosis.

A prospective study randomly assigned 52 patients with HCV-associated type II cryoglobulinemia either to receive interferon alfa or to a control group.[61] Patients with decompensated liver disease were excluded. Fifteen of 25 patients in the treatment group, but none of the control subjects, had undetectable HCV viral loads at the end of the 24-week treatment period. Virologic response was associated with decreases in cryoglobulins, rheumatoid factor, and serum creatinine and an increase in complement levels.

Fourteen patients with MPGN and HCV infection (mostly chronic active hepatitis on liver biopsy) received interferon alfa for 6 to 12 months.[62] Among virologic responders, there was a significant fall in proteinuria, but no improvement in serum creatinine values.

In another report, 18 patients with HCV infection, mixed cryoglobulinemia, nephrotic-range proteinuria, and biopsy-proven MPGN were treated with pegylated interferon alfa and ribavirin for a mean of 18 months.[63] HCV viremia clearance was achieved in 12 of 18 patients and was associated with a reduction in cryoglobulinemia and proteinuria, but serum creatinine levels remained stable regardless of virologic response.

Patients with decreased GFR are at risk for hemolytic anemia when taking ribavirin,[64] and this drug should generally be avoided when creatinine clearance is less than 50 mL/min.

In a recent report, rituximab was successfully used to treat type II cryoglobulinemia and MPGN in patients with HCV infection.[65]

Hepatitis B virus infection

Hepatitis B virus infection is associated with membranous nephropathy, MPGN, and polyarteriitis nodosa. The frequency of HBV-associated glomerulonephritis is greater in endemic areas and may be related to more frequent HBV infection in childhood, leading to a chronic carrier state.[66,67]

Renal deposition of HBV antigens, including HBsAg and HBeAg, suggests an etiologic role of HBV infection in the development of glomerular disease.[67,68]

Membranous nephropathy often presents as nephrotic-range proteinuria or nephrotic syndrome. Biopsy is required to make the diagnosis.

Spontaneous remissions are frequent with HBV-associated membranous nephropathy in children, but the disease has a more progressive course in adults. In a report from China, 21 adult patients with HBV-associated membranous nephropathy were followed up for a mean of 60 months.[67] Progressive renal failure was seen in 29% of the patients, and 10% required hemodialysis at the end of the follow-up.

No randomized clinical trials have been conducted on the treatment of HBV-associated renal disease. Several retrospective reports of antiviral therapy in this setting are presented here. There are no data specifically addressing treatment of HBV-associated glomerular disease in cirrhosis.

In one report, 15 patients with HBV infection and glomerulonephritis (membranous nephropathy or MPGN) were treated with interferon alfa for 6 weeks.[69] Eight patients had a long-term virologic response including disappearance of HBeAg and HBV DNA. Of the responders, 7 showed a gradual improvement in proteinuria during follow-up. All responders had membranous nephropathy. In contrast, the 7 nonresponders continued to have signs of active renal disease; in 1 case there was progression to ESRD. Four of 7 nonresponders had MPGN.

In another report, 10 patients with HBV infection and membranous nephropathy were treated with lamivudine.[70] Outcomes of this report were compared with outcomes in 12 historical controls that had not received antiviral therapy. Blood pressure was well controlled in both groups. Only 1 patient in the treatment group had sonographic evidence of cirrhosis. Lamivudine was associated with significant improvement in proteinuria and clearance of HBsAg. Three-year renal survival was 100% in the antiviral treatment group and 58% in the control group.

Acute Tubular Necrosis

ATN develops in response to nephrotoxic exposures (eg, aminoglycosides, radiocontrast media exposure) or ischemic insult (eg, septic or hemorrhagic shock). Classically, ATN is characterized by acute renal failure following insult, decreased tubular sodium avidity (FeNa > 2%), and muddy-brown casts on microscopic examination of urinary sediment. However, occasionally patients with HRS may have elevated urinary Na^+,[71] and conversely, as a result of high sodium avidity, cirrhotic patients with ATN may have low urinary Na^+.[22]

Postrenal Causes

Common causes of obstructive uropathy include benign prostatic hypertrophy, neurogenic bladder, and kidney stones. In some reports, renal papillary necrosis was associated with alcoholic liver disease.[72,73] Renal imaging (ultrasound, CT scanning) can help detect hydronephrosis or urinary retention. Treatment of renal failure should focus on relieving obstruction.

Medications

Nonsteroidal antiinflammatory drugs

Renal perfusion in patients with liver cirrhosis is highly dependent on vasodilatory effects of prostaglandins, especially prostaglandin E_2 and prostacyclin.[74] NSAIDs inhibit synthesis of prostaglandins and may cause a transient decrease in GFR and impairment in sodium and water excretion in patients with cirrhosis.[75,76] NSAIDs can also cause ascites to become resistant to diuretics.[77] For these reasons, the use of NSAIDs should generally be avoided in patients with liver cirrhosis.

Inhibitors of the renin-angiotensin-aldosterone system

Angiotensin-converting enzyme inhibitors and angiotensin receptor blockers should be used with caution in patients with cirrhosis and are rarely used in patients with advanced liver disease because they may cause hypotension.[78] Angiotensin II helps maintain GFR in cirrhotic patients with decreased renal perfusion by mediating efferent arteriolar constriction. ACE inhibitors or angiotensin receptor blockers, even at low doses that have no effect on systemic blood pressure, may cause a significant reduction in GFR and worsening of sodium retention in patients with cirrhosis.[78]

Aminoglycosides

Aminoglycoside antibiotics are a well-known cause of toxic tubular injury. Clinical records of 214 patients receiving gentamicin or tobramycin were reviewed, and liver disease was found to be one of the risk factors of renal failure with aminoglycoside use.[79] In another retrospective case-control study of US veterans with cirrhosis, aminoglycoside use was strongly associated with acute renal failure.[80]

RENAL REPLACEMENT THERAPY IN CIRRHOSIS

Patients with advanced cirrhosis and renal failure undergoing hemodialysis are prone to intradialytic hypotension due to decreased EABV and higher risk of bleeding with anticoagulation.[81,82]

Despite difficulties and high patient mortality, RRT is an important bridge to liver transplantation. According to 1 retrospective review of 102 liver transplant candidates undergoing acute RRT, 35% survived to receive liver transplant.[83] The 1-year mortality of patients requiring RRT before liver transplantation, however, was 30%, compared with 9.7% for other liver recipients.

Peritoneal dialysis may be better tolerated hemodynamically and no anticoagulation is required. In addition, ascites fluid may be directly removed via peritoneal dialysis catheter, obviating the need for LVP. Potential concerns include higher incidence of peritonitis, protein loss, and bleeding during catheter insertion. In 1 report, 9 patients with ESRD, chronic liver disease, and ascites were initiated on peritoneal dialysis.[84] No complications occurred from catheter insertion, peritonitis rates were similar to patients on peritoneal dialysis without cirrhosis, and serum albumin levels remained stable in most patients. Another report comparing peritoneal dialysis outcomes in 21 cirrhotic patients and 41 patients without cirrhosis did not show a significant difference in the rate of peritonitis.[85] Serum albumin remained steady in patients with cirrhosis. Five-year patient and technique survival rates were similar in both groups.

Simultaneous Liver-Kidney Transplantation

Pretransplant renal function is a strong predictor of both short- and long-term survival in liver transplant recipients.[15] To improve prognosis in patients with dual organ failure, simultaneous liver-kidney transplantation (SLK) should be considered. A recent consensus conference addressed the complex issue of SLK.[86] The following groups are granted automatic approval for SLK transplantation:

- Patients with ESRD who have cirrhosis and symptomatic portal hypertension or hepatic vein wedge pressure with gradient of 10 mm Hg or more
- Patients who have end-stage liver disease (ESLD) and chronic kidney disease with GFR of 30 mL/min or less
- Patients who have acute kidney injury (including HRS) with creatinine 2 mg/dL or more that have been on dialysis for 8 weeks or more
- Patients with ESLD and chronic kidney disease who have greater than 30% glomerulosclerosis or 30% fibrosis on kidney biopsy

Online registry for SLK has been established to monitor patient outcomes and help further redefine the criteria for SLK transplantation.

REFERENCES

1. Stevens LA, Levey AS. Measurement of kidney function. Med Clin North Am 2005; 89(3):457–73.
2. Cocchetto DM, Tschanz C, Bjornsson TD. Decreased rate of creatinine production in patients with hepatic disease: implications for estimation of creatinine clearance. Ther Drug Monit 1983;5(2):161–8.
3. Sherman DS, Fish DN, Teitelbaum I. Assessing renal function in cirrhotic patients: problems and pitfalls. Am J Kidney Dis 2003;41(2):269–78.
4. Roy L, Legault L, Pomier-Layrargues G. Glomerular filtration rate measurement in cirrhotic patients with renal failure. Clin Nephrol 1998;50(6):342–6.
5. Papadakis MA, Arieff AI. Unpredictability of clinical evaluation of renal function in cirrhosis. Prospective study. Am J Med 1987;82(5):945–52.
6. Gonwa TA, Jennings L, Mai ML, et al. Estimation of glomerular filtration rates before and after orthotopic liver transplantation: evaluation of current equations. Liver Transpl 2004;10(2):301–9.
7. Orlando R, Mussap M, Plebani M, et al. Diagnostic value of plasma cystatin C as a glomerular filtration marker in decompensated liver cirrhosis. Clin Chem 2002; 48(6 Pt 1):850–8.
8. Poge U, Gerhardt T, Stoffel-Wagner B, et al. Calculation of glomerular filtration rate based on cystatin C in cirrhotic patients. Nephrol Dial Transplant 2006; 21(3):660–4.
9. Cholongitas E, Marelli L, Kerry A, et al. Different methods of creatinine measurement significantly affect MELD scores. Liver Transpl 2007;13(4):523–9.
10. Daugherty NA, Hammond KB, Osberg IM. Bilirubin interference with the kinetic Jaffe method for serum creatinine. Clin Chem 1978;24(2):392–3.
11. Malinchoc M, Kamath PS, Gordon FD, et al. A model to predict poor survival in patients undergoing transjugular intrahepatic portosystemic shunts. Hepatology 2000;31(4):864–71.

12. Wiesner R, Edwards E, Freeman R, et al. Model for end-stage liver disease (MELD) and allocation of donor livers. Gastroenterology 2003;124(1):91–6.

13. United Network for Organ Sharing. Resources: MELD/PELD calculator. Available at: http://www.unos.org/resources/MeldPeldCalculator.asp?index=98. Accessed November 17, 2008.

14. Alessandria C, Ozdogan O, Guevara M, et al. MELD score and clinical type predict prognosis in hepatorenal syndrome: relevance to liver transplantation. Hepatology 2005;41(6):1282–9.

15. Nair S, Verma S, Thuluvath PJ. Pretransplant renal function predicts survival in patients undergoing orthotopic liver transplantation. Hepatology 2002;35(5):1179–85.

16. Martin PY, Gines P, Schrier RW. Nitric oxide as a mediator of hemodynamic abnormalities and sodium and water retention in cirrhosis. N Engl J Med 1998;339(8):533–41.

17. Schrier RW, Arroyo V, Bernardi M, et al. Peripheral arterial vasodilation hypothesis: a proposal for the initiation of renal sodium and water retention in cirrhosis. Hepatology 1988;8(5):1151–7.

18. Arroyo V, Bosch J, Gaya-Beltran J, et al. Plasma renin activity and urinary sodium excretion as prognostic indicators in nonazotemic cirrhosis with ascites. Ann Intern Med 1981;94(2):198–201.

19. Bichet DG, Van Putten VJ, Schrier RW. Potential role of increased sympathetic activity in impaired sodium and water excretion in cirrhosis. N Engl J Med 1982;307(25):1552–7.

20. Bichet D, Szatalowicz V, Chaimovitz C, et al. Role of vasopressin in abnormal water excretion in cirrhotic patients. Ann Intern Med 1982;96(4):413–7.

21. Pockros PJ, Reynolds TB. Rapid diuresis in patients with ascites from chronic liver disease: the importance of peripheral edema. Gastroenterology 1986;90(6):1827–33.

22. Arroyo V, Gines P, Gerbes AL, et al. Definition and diagnostic criteria of refractory ascites and hepatorenal syndrome in cirrhosis. International Ascites Club. Hepatology 1996;23(1):164–76.

23. Gines P, Tito L, Arroyo V, et al. Randomized comparative study of therapeutic paracentesis with and without intravenous albumin in cirrhosis. Gastroenterology 1988;94(6):1493–502.

24. Runyon BA. Management of adult patients with ascites due to cirrhosis. Hepatology 2004;39(3):841–56.

25. Gines A, Escorsell A, Gines P, et al. Incidence, predictive factors, and prognosis of the hepatorenal syndrome in cirrhosis with ascites. Gastroenterology 1993;105(1):229–36.

26. Fernandez-Seara J, Prieto J, Quiroga J, et al. Systemic and regional hemodynamics in patients with liver cirrhosis and ascites with and without functional renal failure. Gastroenterology 1989;97(5):1304–12.

27. Ruiz-del-Arbol L, Monescillo A, Arocena C, et al. Circulatory function and hepatorenal syndrome in cirrhosis. Hepatology 2005;42(2):439–47.

28. Follo A, Llovet JM, Navasa M, et al. Renal impairment after spontaneous bacterial peritonitis in cirrhosis: incidence, clinical course, predictive factors and prognosis. Hepatology 1994;20(6):1495–501.

29. Salerno F, Gerbes A, Gines P, et al. Diagnosis, prevention and treatment of hepatorenal syndrome in cirrhosis. Gut 2007;56(9):1310–8.

30. Sort P, Navasa M, Arroyo V, et al. Effect of intravenous albumin on renal impairment and mortality in patients with cirrhosis and spontaneous bacterial peritonitis. N Engl J Med 1999;341(6):403–9.

31. Fernandez J, Navasa M, Planas R, et al. Primary prophylaxis of spontaneous bacterial peritonitis delays hepatorenal syndrome and improves survival in cirrhosis. Gastroenterology 2007;133(3):818–24.

32. Angeli P, Volpin R, Gerunda G, et al. Reversal of type 1 hepatorenal syndrome with the administration of midodrine and octreotide. Hepatology 1999;29(6):1690–7.

33. Martin-Llahi M, Pepin MN, Guevara M, et al. Terlipressin and albumin vs albumin in patients with cirrhosis and hepatorenal syndrome: a randomized study. Gastroenterology 2008;134(5):1352–9.

34. Sanyal AJ, Boyer T, Garcia-Tsao G, et al. A randomized, prospective, double-blind, placebo-controlled trial of terlipressin for type 1 hepatorenal syndrome. Gastroenterology 2008;134(5):1360–8.

35. Duvoux C, Zanditenas D, Hezode C, et al. Effects of noradrenalin and albumin in patients with type I hepatorenal syndrome: a pilot study. Hepatology 2002;36(2):374–80.

36. Munoz SJ. The hepatorenal syndrome. Med Clin North Am 2008;92(4):813–37, viii–ix.

37. Lim JK, Groszmann RJ. Vasoconstrictor therapy for the hepatorenal syndrome. Gastroenterology 2008;134(5):1608–11.

38. Gonwa TA, Morris CA, Goldstein RM, et al. Long-term survival and renal function following liver transplantation in patients with and without hepatorenal syndrome–experience in 300 patients. Transplantation 1991;51(2):428–30.

39. de Cleva R, Silva FP, Zilberstein B, et al. Acute renal failure due to abdominal compartment syndrome: report on four cases and literature review. Rev Hosp Clin Fac Med Sao Paulo 2001;56(4):123–30.

40. Cheatham ML, Malbrain ML, Kirkpatrick A, et al. Results from the International Conference of Experts on Intra-abdominal Hypertension and Abdominal Compartment Syndrome. II. Recommendations. Intensive Care Med 2007;33(6):951–62.

41. Richards WO, Scovill W, Shin B, et al. Acute renal failure associated with increased intra-abdominal pressure. Ann Surg 1983;197(2):183–7.

42. Doty JM, Saggi BH, Blocher CR, et al. Effects of increased renal parenchymal pressure on renal function. J Trauma 2000;48(5):874–7.

43. Sugrue M, Bauman A, Jones F, et al. Clinical examination is an inaccurate predictor of intraabdominal pressure. World J Surg 2002;26(12):1428–31.

44. Sinniah R. Heterogeneous IgA glomerulonephropathy in liver cirrhosis. Histopathology 1984;8(6):947–62.

45. McGuire BM, Julian BA, Bynon JSJ, et al. Brief communication: Glomerulonephritis in patients with hepatitis C cirrhosis undergoing liver transplantation. Ann Intern Med 2006;144(10):735–41.

46. Sancho J, Egido J, Sanchez-Crespo M, et al. Detection of monomeric and polymeric IgA containing immune complexes in serum and kidney from patients with alcoholic liver disease. Clin Exp Immunol 1982;47(2):327–35.

47. Coppo R, Arico S, Piccoli G, et al. Presence and origin of IgA1- and IgA2-containing circulating immune complexes in chronic alcoholic liver diseases with and without glomerulonephritis. Clin Immunol Immunopathol 1985;35(1):1–8.

48. Giron JA, Alvarez-Mon M, Menendez-Caro JL, et al. Increased spontaneous and lymphokine-conditioned IgA and IgG synthesis by B cells from alcoholic cirrhotic patients. Hepatology 1992;16(3):664–70.

49. Delacroix DL, Elkom KB, Geubel AP, et al. Changes in size, subclass, and metabolic properties of serum immunoglobulin A in liver diseases and in other diseases with high serum immunoglobulin A. J Clin Invest 1983;71(2):358–67.

50. Rifai A, Fadden K, Morrison SL, et al. The N-glycans determine the differential blood clearance and hepatic uptake of human immunoglobulin (Ig)A1 and IgA2 isotypes. J Exp Med 2000;191(12):2171–82.

51. Lomax-Smith JD, Zabrowarny LA, Howarth GS, et al. The immunochemical characterization of mesangial IgA deposits. Am J Pathol 1983;113(3):359–64.

52. Kalambokis G, Christou L, Stefanou D, et al. Association of liver cirrhosis related IgA nephropathy with portal hypertension. World J Gastroenterol 2007;13(43):5783–6.

53. Nakamura M, Ohishi A, Watanabe R, et al. IgA nephropathy associated with portal hypertension in liver cirrhosis due to non-alcoholic and non-A, non-B, non-C hepatitis. Intern Med 1994;33(8):488–91.

54. Arase Y, Ikeda K, Murashima N, et al. Glomerulonephritis in autopsy cases with hepatitis C virus infection. Intern Med 1998;37(10):836–40.

55. Johnson RJ, Willson R, Yamabe H, et al. Renal manifestations of hepatitis C virus infection. Kidney Int 1994;46(5):1255–63.

56. Agnello V, Chung RT, Kaplan LM. A role for hepatitis C virus infection in type II cryoglobulinemia. N Engl J Med 1992;327(21):1490–5.

57. Uchiyama-Tanaka Y, Mori Y, Kishimoto N, et al. Membranous glomerulonephritis associated with hepatitis C virus infection: case report and literature review. Clin Nephrol 2004;61(2):144–50.

58. Stehman-Breen C, Alpers CE, Couser WG, et al. Hepatitis C virus associated membranous glomerulonephritis. Clin Nephrol 1995;44(3):141–7.

59. Altraif IH, Abdulla AS, al Sebayel MI, et al. Hepatitis C associated glomerulonephritis. Am J Nephrol 1995;15(5):407–10.

60. Sansonno D, Gesualdo L, Manno C, et al. Hepatitis C virus-related proteins in kidney tissue from hepatitis C virus-infected patients with cryoglobulinemic membranoproliferative glomerulonephritis. Hepatology 1997;25(5):1237–44.

61. Misiani R, Bellavita P, Fenili D, et al. Interferon alfa-2a therapy in cryoglobulinemia associated with hepatitis C virus. N Engl J Med 1994;330(11):751–6.

62. Johnson RJ, Gretch DR, Couser WG, et al. Hepatitis C virus-associated glomerulonephritis. Effect of alpha-interferon therapy. Kidney Int 1994;46(6):1700–4.

63. Alric L, Plaisier E, Thebault S, et al. Influence of antiviral therapy in hepatitis C virus-associated cryoglobulinemic MPGN. Am J Kidney Dis 2004;43(4):617–23.

64. Reau N, Hadziyannis SJ, Messinger D, et al. Early predictors of anemia in patients with hepatitis C genotype 1 treated with peginterferon alfa-2a (40KD) plus ribavirin. Am J Gastroenterol 2008;103(8):1981–8.

65. Roccatello D, Baldovino S, Rossi D, et al. Long-term effects of anti-CD20 monoclonal antibody treatment of cryoglobulinaemic glomerulonephritis. Nephrol Dial Transplant 2004;19(12):3054–61.

66. Levy M, Chen N. Worldwide perspective of hepatitis B-associated glomerulonephritis in the 80s. Kidney Int Suppl 1991;35:S24–33.

67. Lai KN, Li PK, Lui SF, et al. Membranous nephropathy related to hepatitis B virus in adults. N Engl J Med 1991;324(21):1457–63.

68. Takekoshi Y, Tochimaru H, Nagata Y, et al. Immunopathogenetic mechanisms of hepatitis B virus-related glomerulopathy. Kidney Int Suppl 1991;35:S34–9.

69. Conjeevaram HS, Hoofnagle JH, Austin HA, et al. Long-term outcome of hepatitis B virus-related glomerulonephritis after therapy with interferon alfa. Gastroenterology 1995;109(2):540–6.

70. Tang S, Lai FM, Lui YH, et al. Lamivudine in hepatitis B-associated membranous nephropathy. Kidney Int 2005;68(4):1750–8.

71. Dudley FJ, Kanel GC, Wood LJ, et al. Hepatorenal syndrome without avid sodium retention. Hepatology 1986;6(2):248–51.

72. Edmondson HA, Reynolds TB, Jacobson HG. Renal papillary necrosis with special reference to chronic alcoholism. A report of 20 cases. Arch Intern Med 1966;118(3):255–64.
73. Longacre AM, Popky GL. Papillary necrosis in patients with cirrhosis: a study of 102 patients. J Urol 1968;99(4):391–5.
74. Lopez-Parra M, Claria J, Planaguma A, et al. Cyclooxygenase-1 derived prostaglandins are involved in the maintenance of renal function in rats with cirrhosis and ascites. Br J Pharmacol 2002;135(4):891–900.
75. Hsia HC, Lin HC, Tsai YT, et al. The effects of chronic administration of indomethacin and misoprostol on renal function in cirrhotic patients with and without ascites. Scand J Gastroenterol 1995;30(12):1194–9.
76. Brater DC, Anderson SA, Brown-Cartwright D, et al. Effects of nonsteroidal anti-inflammatory drugs on renal function in patients with renal insufficiency and in cirrhotics. Am J Kidney Dis 1986;8(5):351–5.
77. Runyon BA. Refractory ascites. Semin Liver Dis 1993;13(4):343–51.
78. Henriksen JH, Moller S. Liver cirrhosis and arterial hypertension. World J Gastroenterol 2006;12(5):678–85.
79. Moore RD, Smith CR, Lipsky JJ, et al. Risk factors for nephrotoxicity in patients treated with aminoglycosides. Ann Intern Med 1984;100(3):352–7.
80. Hampel H, Bynum GD, Zamora E, et al. Risk factors for the development of renal dysfunction in hospitalized patients with cirrhosis. Am J Gastroenterol 2001;96(7):2206–10.
81. Howard CS, Teitelbaum I. Renal replacement therapy in patients with chronic liver disease. Semin Dial 2005;18(3):212–6.
82. Wilkinson SP, Weston MJ, Parsons V, et al. Dialysis in the treatment of renal failure in patients with liver disease. Clin Nephrol 1977;8(1):287–92.
83. Wong LP, Blackley MP, Andreoni KA, et al. Survival of liver transplant candidates with acute renal failure receiving renal replacement therapy. Kidney Int 2005;68(1):362–70.
84. Marcus RG, Messana J, Swartz R. Peritoneal dialysis in end-stage renal disease patients with preexisting chronic liver disease and ascites. Am J Med 1992;93(1):35–40.
85. De Vecchi AF, Colucci P, Salerno F, et al. Outcome of peritoneal dialysis in cirrhotic patients with chronic renal failure. Am J Kidney Dis 2002;40(1):161–8.
86. Eason JD, Gonwa TA, Davis CL, et al. Proceedings of Consensus Conference on Simultaneous Liver Kidney Transplantation (SLK). Am J Transplant 2008;8(11):2243–51.

Pulmonary Complications of Cirrhosis

C. Singh, MD[a], J.S. Sager, MD, MSc[b],*

KEYWORDS

- Pulmonary hypertension • Hepatopulmonary syndrome
- Portopulmonary hypertension • Hepatic hydrothorax
- Liver transplantation

"Is life worth living? It all depends on the liver."
William James, American philosopher (1842)

The liver is the gatekeeper of physiologic homeostasis, and disruption of this homeostasis leads to multiorgan dysfunction. Cirrhosis is the twelfth leading cause of death and accounts for 1.1% of all deaths in the United States.[1] This issue of *The Medical Clinics of North America* is an extensive review of hepatic disease and its devastating effects on organ systems.

Pulmonary manifestations and complications of liver disease are numerous, and this article reviews 3 of the most common complications, namely hepatopulmonary syndrome (HPS), portopulmonary hypertension (POPH), and hepatic hydrothorax.

The autoimmune liver diseases, primary biliary cirrhosis and autoimmune hepatitis, may be accompanied by immune-mediated lung disease.[2] Other important pulmonary manifestations of cirrhosis are susceptibility to pneumonia and restrictive lung physiology related to diaphragmatic elevation because of massive ascites.[2] Pulmonary complications of liver cirrhosis cause significant morbidity and affect patients' quality of life.

HEPATOPULMONARY SYNDROME

The term *hepatopulmonary syndrome* was first coined by Kennedy and Knudson in 1977.[3] HPS is characterized by decreased systemic arterial oxygenation induced by pulmonary vascular dilation associated with liver disease (**Table 1**). The clinical triad

[a] Santa Barbara Cottage Hospital, 675 Central Avenue, Apartment 5, Buellton, CA 93427, USA
[b] Cottage Pulmonary Hypertension Center, Keck School of Medicine, University of Southern California, 2403 Castillo Street, Suite 206, Santa Barbara, CA 93105, USA
* Corresponding author.
E-mail address: jsager@sblung.com (J.S. Sager).

Med Clin N Am 93 (2009) 871–883
doi:10.1016/j.mcna.2009.03.006
0025-7125/09/$ – see front matter © 2009 Elsevier Inc. All rights reserved.

Table 1
Distinction between hepatopulmonary syndrome and portopulmonary hypertension

	HPS	PPHTN
Symptomatology	Progressive dyspnea	Progressive dyspnea Chest pain Syncope
Clinical examination	Cyanosis Finger clubbing Spider angiomas (?)	No cyanosis RV heave Pronounced P2 component
ECG findings	None	RBBB Rightward axis RV hypertrophy
Arterial blood gas levels	Moderate to severe hypoxemia	No/mild hypoxemia
Chest radiography	Normal	Cardiomegaly Hilar enlargement
CEE	Always positive; left atrial opacification for >3–6 cardiac cycles after right atrial opacification	Usually negative; however, positive for <3 cardiac cycles (if atrial septal defect or patent foramen ovale exists)
^{99m}TcMAA shunting index	$\geq$6%	<6%
Pulmonary hemodynamics	Normal/low PVR	Elevated PVR Normal mPAP
Pulmonary angiography	Normal/"spongy" appearance (type I) Discrete AV communications (type II)	Large main pulmonary arteries Distal arterial pruning
OLT	Always indicated in severe stages	Only indicated in mild to moderate stages

Data from Rodriguez-Roisin R, Krowka MJ, Herve P, Fallon MB. Pulmonary hepatic-vascular disorders (PHD). Eur Respir J 2004;24(5):873.

of HPS includes an elevated room air alveolar-arterial (A-a) gradient, liver disease, and evidence of intrapulmonary vascular dilatation (IPVD).

The prevalence of HPS ranges from 5% to 32%.[4] Various ranges of abnormal A-a gradient and partial pressure of oxygen (Po_2) used to define gas exchange issues lead to the range in prevalence of HPS.

The median survival for HPS without liver transplant is 24 months with a 5-year survival rate of about 23%.[5] Schiffer and colleagues[6] recently described that the presence of HPS worsened the prognosis for patients with cirrhosis, even after adjusting for the Child classification of liver disease. Worse survival is evident if the presenting Po_2 is less than 50 mm Hg; however, death caused by severe hypoxemic respiratory failure is rare in HPS and is usually associated with complications of the hepatic disease.[7]

Pathophysiology

IPVD is thought to be the major cause for severe hypoxemia related to HPS.[8] A number of postulates have been proposed.

1. Failure of the damaged liver to clear pulmonary vasodilators (intestinal endotoxemia).[9]

2. Production of circulatory vasodilators by the damaged liver. These include vasodilator prostaglandins (such as prostacyclin, prostaglandin E_1, and prostaglandin I_2), nitric oxide (NO), vasoactive intestinal peptide, calcitonin, and glucagon. Substance P, atrial natriuretic factor, and platelet-activating factor are additional potent vasodilators that are elevated in hepatic disease.[10,11] NO plays a major role in HPS animal models. Upregulation of endothelial nitric oxide synthase (eNOS) in the pulmonary arteries and NO-mediated impairment of phenylephrine-induced vasoconstriction lead to HPS in rats.[12]

3. Enhanced eNOS-derived NO production may result from pulmonary endothelial endothelin B (ETB)–receptor overexpression and increased circulating endothelin-1 (ET-1)–induced vasodilation.[13]

These findings are consistent with observations that exhaled NO levels are increased and administration of NO inhibitors (eg, methylene blue) can enhance oxygenation in patients with HPS.[14–17]

Pulmonary Vascular Shunting

The unique pathologic feature of HPS is dilation of the pulmonary precapillary and capillary vessels. Supplemental oxygen enhances oxygenation more than expected with true "anatomic" shunts; a new mechanism has been invoked to explain the hypoxemia associated with HPS. This mechanism has been called diffusion-perfusion impairment or alveolar-capillary oxygen disequilibrium.[18–20] Diffusion-perfusion impairment relates to the mechanism of hypoxemia associated with IPVD. Because the capillary is dilated and has an expanded diameter, oxygen molecules from adjacent alveoli cannot diffuse to the center of the dilated vessel to oxygenate hemoglobin in the erythrocytes in the center stream of venous blood.[21] Supplemental oxygen provides enough driving pressure to partially overcome this relative diffusion defect. In HPS many capillaries are dilated and blood flow is not uniform. Ventilation-perfusion defects are the predominant mechanisms and coexist with restricted oxygen diffusion into the center of dilated capillaries in advanced stages (**Fig. 1**).[7,22]

In the context of a diffusion-like impairment of oxygenation in HPS, oxygenation is further limited by the increased cardiac output associated with liver disease, which reduces the transit time through the lung vasculature and the amount of time available for oxygen diffusion.[8,23] Thorens and Junod[24] demonstrated the effect of this shortened transit time by showing that exercise in a patient with cirrhosis who was breathing 100% oxygen caused further impairment of oxygenation and development of a large shunt fraction.

Clinical Manifestations

Unique features of HPS are the platypnea, defined as dyspnea induced by the upright position and relieved by a recumbent position, and orthodeoxia, defined as arterial deoxygenation induced by upright position and relieved by reclining. Although these phenomena are not pathognomonic for HPS, in liver dysfunction they strongly suggest HPS.[25,26]

Dyspnea with exertion is the most common symptom. The presence of spider nevi, cyanosis, digital clubbing, and severe hypoxemia point strongly toward HPS.[27]

Most patients with HPS will present with signs and symptoms of liver disease, including gastrointestinal bleeding, esophageal varices, ascites, palmar erythema, and splenomegaly.[28]

The chest radiograph is often nonspecific with increased markings at the bases that may reflect diffuse vascular pulmonary dilation.[7]

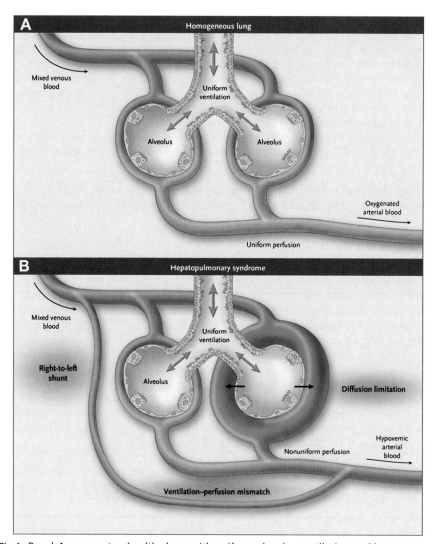

Fig. 1. Panel *A* represents a healthy lung with uniform alveolar ventilation and homogenous blood flow. Panel *B* shows 2 major reasons for shunting, namely ventilation-perfusion mismatch and vascular dilation with diffusion limitation. (*From* Rodriguez-Roisin R, Krowka MJ. Hepatopulmonary syndrome—a liver-induced lung vascular disorder. N Engl J Med 2008;358(22):2384; with permission.)

A decrease in the diffusion capacity for carbon monoxide on pulmonary function testing is consistently abnormal in patients with HPS and may not improve even after liver transplantation.[29,30]

Diagnosis

Contrast enhanced echocardiography is a valuable tool for showing the presence and prevalence of IPVD in patients with hypoxemia and liver disease. This is the preferred diagnostic modality for diagnosing IPVDs.[31,32] Microbubble opacification of the left atrium within 3 to 6 cardiac cycles after right atrial opacification indicates microbubble passage through an abnormally dilated pulmonary vascular bed. Microbubbles do not pass through normal capillary diameter.

Nuclear lung scanning using technetium-labeled macroaggregated albumin showing the uptake of radionucleotide in brain and kidney suggests shunt with transit through intrapulmonary vessels.[31]

Pulmonary angiography is indicated only when hypoxemia is severe (P_{O_2} is <60 mm Hg) to evaluate for pulmonary arteriovenous malformations that would be amenable to percutaneous embolization.[33]

There are 2 radiographic patterns distinguished on pulmonary angiography:

Type 1—Minimal pattern characterized by normal to finely diffuse, spidery abnormalities with good response to 100% inspired oxygen.

Type 2—Discrete pattern characterized by localized arteriovenous (AV) communications, poor response to supplemental oxygen.

Shunt study: The arterial P_{O_2} is measured with the patient first breathing room air and then breathing 100% oxygen in the supine and standing positions. If the arterial P_{O_2} on 100% oxygen is less than 200 mm Hg, severe dilatations, discrete AV communications, or intracardiac shunt should be suspected.

Diagnostic Criteria for HPS

1. P_{O_2} less than 80 mm Hg or A-a gradient more than 15 mm Hg on room air.[7]
2. Positive finding on contrast enhanced echocardiography or abnormal uptake in the brain with radioactive lung perfusion scan.
3. Portal hypertension with or without cirrhosis.

Treatment

Currently there are no effective medical therapies for HPS, with liver transplant being the only effective surgical treatment. Spontaneous resolution of HPS is rare and treatment attempts using antibiotics, β-blockade, steroids, cyclophosphamide, inhaled NO, and NO inhibitors have shown no benefit in uncontrolled trials.[27]

Liver Transplant

HPS can reverse after liver transplantation despite the presence of hypoxemia. However, postoperative mortality increases in patients with significant pretransplant hypoxemia related to HPS.[34] HPS is a clear and definitive indication for liver transplant. United Network for Organ Sharing policy 3.6.4.5.1 provides exception points for patients diagnosed with HPS to compensate for their increased mortality risk.[27,35]

In the Mayo Clinic series, patients with HPS have a 5-year survival rate of 76% after liver transplant, similar to posttransplant patients without HPS. The strongest predictor of death was preoperative P_{O_2} of 50 mm Hg or less and lung scan with brain uptake of 20% or more.[5] Patients with P_{O_2} of 60 mm Hg or less should be considered candidates for liver transplant and given priority for liver transplantation.[7]

PORTOPULMONARY HYPERTENSION

POPH is defined as the development of pulmonary arterial hypertension associated with increased pulmonary vascular resistance (PVR) complicated by portal hypertension with or without advanced hepatic disease. This means an increase in mean pulmonary arterial pressure (mPAP) more than 25 mm Hg in the setting of portal hypertension.[27]

POPH was first described by Mantz and Craige in 1951;[36] since then the disease continues to receive increased attention because of its significant implication for appropriate candidacy for liver transplant.

POPH is classified as a subset of pulmonary arterial hypertension (**Table 2**).

A classification of the severity of POPH was proposed in 2004, according to which mild disease has mPAP of 24 to 34 mm Hg, moderate disease mPAP ranges from 35 to 44 mm Hg, and severe disease has an mPAP of 45 mm Hg and higher.[37]

Epidemiology

The prevalence of POPH in patients with liver disease is not well defined. Older studies showed that the prevalence of pulmonary artery hypertension ranged from 0.25% to

Table 2
Revised clinical classification of pulmonary hypertension (Venice 2003)
1. Pulmonary arterial hypertension (PAH)
1.1. Idiopathic (IPAH)
1.2. Familial (FPAH)
1.3. Associated with (APAH):
1.3.1. Collagen vascular disease
1.3.2. Congenital systemic to pulmonary shunts
1.3.3. Portal hypertension
1.3.4. HIV infection
1.3.5. Drugs and toxins
1.3.6. Other (thyroid disorders, glycogen storage disease, Gaucher disease, hereditary hemorrhagic telangiectasia, hemoglobinopathies, myeloproliferative disorders, splenectomy)
1.4. Associated with significant venous or capillary involvement
1.4.1. Pulmonary venoocclusive disease (PVOD)
1.4.2. Pulmonary capillary hemangiomatosis (PCH)
1.5. Persistent pulmonary hypertension of the newborn
2. Pulmonary hypertension with left heart disease
2.1. Left-sided atrial or ventricular heart disease
2.2. Left-sided valvular heart disease
3. Pulmonary hypertension associated with lung diseases and/or hypoxemia
3.1. Chronic obstructive pulmonary disease
3.2. Interstitial lung disease
3.3. Sleep-disordered breathing
3.4. Alveolar hypoventilation disorders
3.5. Chronic exposure to high altitude
3.6. Developmental abnormalities
4. Pulmonary hypertension because of chronic thrombotic and/or embolic disease
4.1. Thromboembolic obstruction of proximal pulmonary arteries
4.2. Thromboembolic obstruction of distal pulmonary arteries
4.3. Nonthrombotic pulmonary embolism (tumor, parasites, foreign material)
5. Miscellaneous: Sarcoidosis, histiocytosis X, lymphangiomatosis, compression of pulmonary vessels (adenopathy, tumor, fibrosing mediastinitis)

Data from Simonneau G, Galie N, Rubin LJ, et al. Clinical classification of pulmonary hypertension. J Am Coll Cardiol 2004;43(12 Suppl):5S–12S.

0.73% in populations with portal hypertension or cirrhosis, although recent hemody-namic studies estimated prevalence of POPH between 2% and 10%.[38–42]

The mean age of presentation of POPH is in the fifth decade, and the male-female ratio is 1.1:1.

Pathogenesis

At the present time, the pathogenesis of POPH is not fully understood.
Multiple mechanisms are associated with development of POPH:

1. Hyperdynamic circulatory state and increase in cardiac output cause increased shear stress on pulmonary circulation; the PVR rises owing to vasoconstriction, progressive pulmonary remodeling, and thrombosis.[43]
2. Factors such as splanchnic volume overload and bowel wall congestion lead to the release of endotoxins and cytokines, including NO, and prostacyclin (causing dila-tion of vessels) and ET-1 and thromboxane (causing constriction of vessels). Hence the imbalance between pulmonary vasodilation and vasoconstriction promotes pulmonary arterial hypertension.[44]
3. Hallmarks of POPH are proliferative pulmonary arteriopathy with formation of plexiform lesions, necrotizing arteritis with fibrinoid necrosis and thrombosis.[45]

Clinical Findings

In early stages of POPH, patients are mostly asymptomatic.

The most common initial symptom is progressive dyspnea on exertion. Other symp-toms such as dyspnea at rest, chest pain, palpitations, and syncope or near syncope are less common.[46,47]

On physical examination, appreciable findings generally depend on the severity of POPH. Variable signs include jaundice, spider telangiectasias, accentuated and split second heart sound, systolic murmur, right ventricular heave, right-sided S3 gallop, jugular vein distension, ascites, and edema of lower extremities due to either decom-pensated cirrhosis or right heart failure.

Diagnosis

Transthoracic Doppler echocardiography (TTE) is a useful noninvasive screening test based on its ability to estimate pulmonary arterial systolic pressure when tricuspid regurgitation is present. The positive predictive value of echocardiography for identi-fying clinically significant pulmonary hypertension is 37.5%, and the negative predic-tive value is 91.9%. Hence echocardiography is useful in excluding POPH for those with mPAP less than 15 mm Hg.

TTE is found to have a sensitivity of 97% and a specificity of 77% in diagnosing pulmonary artery hypertension.[48–50]

Right heart catheterization is the gold standard test for the diagnosis, quantification, and characterization of POPH. Hence patients with apparently elevated pulmonary artery systolic pressure more than 50 mm Hg by echocardiography should undergo invasive assessment by right heart catheterization.[51]

Both chest radiography and ECG are poor screening tools for POPH. Chest radiog-raphy findings of enlarged central pulmonary arteries and right-sided cardiomegaly are nonspecific, as are ECG findings of right axis deviation, right bundle branch block (RBBB), and T wave inversion in anterior leads.

Diagnostic Criteria

Patients are considered to have POPH if they have advanced portal hypertension and:

1. An increased mPAP greater than 25 mm Hg at rest or greater than 30 mm Hg on exercise.
2. Elevated PVR greater than 240 dyne/s/cm.
3. Normal or decreased pulmonary artery wedge pressure less than 15 mm Hg.

Management

At the present time, there are no major long-term studies on the use of pharmacotherapy in POPH.

Prostanoids are effective in the treatment of POPH. Epoprostenol, a prostacyclin analog and potent pulmonary and systemic vasodilator with additional antiplatelet aggregating activity if given via continuous central vein infusion, can significantly improve the pulmonary hemodynamics. In certain liver transplant centers this may facilitate the acceptance onto the transplant list for patients who were denied liver transplant as a result of POPH.[52,53]

Major side effects of epoprostenol are worsening hepatic function and resultant clinical deterioration, splenomegaly, and thrombocytopenia.

Iloprost is an alternate to epoprostenol that in combination with bosentan, an ET-1 receptor antagonist, may extend survival of patients with POPH with recurrent right heart failure.[54,55]

Sildenafil, a lung tissue–selective phosphodiestrase-5 inhibitor, blocks the degradation of NO. In combination with oxygen, sildenafil produces pulmonary vasodilation and helps to maintain the selective pulmonary vasodilation effect of inhaled NO.[56]

Liver Transplant

The presence of POPH increases the risk for perioperative and long-term morbidity and mortality associated with liver transplant. Mortality is directly proportional to mPAP and PVR. Few studies suggest that preoperative mPAP is an independent predictor for mortality, and most transplant centers consider mPAP more than 50 mm Hg to be an absolute contraindication for liver transplantation.[57]

Prognosis

Robalino and Moodie[46] described a 21% 30-month survival (n = 49) in patients with POPH in the pre–orthotopic liver transplantation (OLT) era. Swanson and colleagues[58] documented the Mayo Clinic experience, showing a 28% 5-year survival without OLT (n = 66) and 56% with OLT (n = 28).

Mild POPH does not appear to adversely impact liver transplantation; however, more significant elevations in pulmonary pressures are associated with excessive posttransplantation mortality. Data derived from a large retrospective review and from a multicenter liver transplant database[59] document mortality rates of 60% to 100% for liver transplant recipients with a preoperative mean pulmonary artery pressure of or exceeding 50 mm Hg, 35% to 40% for those with mean pressures between 35 and 50 mm Hg, and 0% to –17% for those with mean pulmonary artery pressure below 35 mm Hg. Most deaths are attributed to progressive right heart failure and usually occur intraoperatively. There are rare reports of improvement in pulmonary hemodynamics after liver transplantation.[60,61]

HEPATIC HYDROTHORAX

Hepatic hydrothorax is defined as a pleural effusion usually greater than 500 mL in patients with cirrhosis and without primary cardiac, pulmonary, or pleural disease.

Pathophysiology

The exact mechanisms of the development of hepatic hydrothorax are unclear, although they may involve passage of ascitic fluid from the peritoneal cavity to the pleural cavity via small diaphragmatic defects on the tendinous portion of the diaphragm, as described by Huang and colleagues.[62]

The negative intrathoracic pressure generated during inspiration facilitates the flow from intra-abdominal cavity to the pleural space.

Clinical Manifestation

Dyspnea, cough, and chest discomfort are prominent but nonspecific symptoms.

Diagnosis

1. Chest radiography is the main modality to diagnose hepatic hydrothorax. Right-sided hydrothorax is present in 85% of patients, left-sided in 15%, and bilateral in 2%.
2. Thoracentesis should be performed to confirm the diagnosis and exclude other causes of pleural effusions, specifically infection or malignancy.
3. CT of chest should be performed to exclude mediastinal, pulmonary, and pleural lesions.
4. Abdominal ultrasonography with Doppler should be performed to examine the liver and ascertain the patency of the portal and hepatic veins.

Management

The most important aspect of management is evaluation for liver transplantation. The primary aim of treatment is relief of symptoms and prevention of pulmonary complications and infections until liver transplant can be performed, or palliative treatment in those who are not transplant candidates.

1. Sodium restriction and diureticsare initial management, as in ascites.
2. Therapeutic thoracentesis is an effective way to reduce large effusions in refractory hydrothorax; however, repeat thoracentesis is not recommended due to albumin depletion and rapid recurrence.
3. Transjugular intrahepatic portosystemic shunt (TIPS) should be considered in selected patients with a Child-Pugh score less than 10, age less than 60 years, and without any evidence of hepatic encephalopathy.[63]
4. Pleurodesis—hepatic hydrothorax is the most difficult form of nonmalignant pleural effusion to treat with chemical pleurodesis, as rapid migration of fluid from abdomen into the pleural space often does not allow for successful pleurodesis. This procedure is reserved as a palliative measure in select patients.
5. Splanchnic vasoconstrictors—limited data is available about successful use of octreotide for refractory hydrothorax. Use of terlipressin has also been described.[64,65]

SUMMARY

In portal hypertension and liver cirrhosis, a wide spectrum of pulmonary complications can occur. This article reviews the diagnosis and management of HPS, POPH, and hepatic hydrothorax. Patients presenting with cirrhosis who are experiencing dyspnea need to be evaluated thoroughly for the above diseases. The development of POPH may be an exclusion criteria for liver transplant in most patients affected, whereas the development of HPS may indeed be an indication for liver transplant. Pulmonary complications of cirrhosis have a significant impact on patient outcomes and morbidity and greatly affect the quality of life of patients suffering from these diseases.

REFERENCES

1. Kung HC, Hoyert DL, Xu J, et al. Deaths: final data for 2005. Natl Vital Stat Rep 2008;56(10):1–120.
2. King PD, Rumbaut R, Sanchez C. Pulmonary manifestations of chronic liver disease. Dig Dis 1996;14(2):73–82.
3. Kennedy TC, Knudson RJ. Exercise-aggravated hypoxemia and orthodeoxia in cirrhosis. Chest 1977;72(3):305–9.
4. Schenk P, Fuhrmann V, Madl C, et al. Hepatopulmonary syndrome: prevalence and predictive value of various cut offs for arterial oxygenation and their clinical consequences. Gut 2002;51(6):853–9.
5. Swanson KL, Wiesner RH, Krowka MJ. Natural history of hepatopulmonary syndrome: impact of liver transplantation. Hepatology 2005;41(5):1122–9.
6. Schiffer E, Majno P, Mentha G, et al. Hepatopulmonary syndrome increases the postoperative mortality rate following liver transplantation: a prospective study in 90 patients. Am J Transplant 2006;6(6):1430–7.
7. Rodriguez-Roisin R, Krowka MJ. Hepatopulmonary syndrome–a liver-induced lung vascular disorder. N Engl J Med 2008;358(22):2378–87.
8. Krowka MJ, Cortese DA. Hepatopulmonary syndrome: an evolving perspective in the era of liver transplantation. Hepatology 1990;11(1):138–42.
9. Zhang HY, Han de W, Su AR, et al. Intestinal endotoxemia plays a central role in development of hepatopulmonary syndrome in a cirrhotic rat model induced by multiple pathogenic factors. World J Gastroenterol 2007;13(47):6385–95.
10. Bruix J, Bosch J, Kravetz D, et al. Effects of prostaglandin inhibition on systemic and hepatic hemodynamics in patients with cirrhosis of the liver. Gastroenterology 1985;88(2):430–5.
11. Zipser RD, Hoefs JC, Speckart PF, et al. Prostaglandins: modulators of renal function and pressor resistance in chronic liver disease. J Clin Endocrinol Metab 1979;48(6):895–900.
12. Fallon MB, Abrams GA, Luo B, et al. The role of endothelial nitric oxide synthase in the pathogenesis of a rat model of hepatopulmonary syndrome. Gastroenterology 1997;113(2):606–14.
13. Tang L, Luo B, Patel RP, et al. Modulation of pulmonary endothelial endothelin B receptor expression and signaling: implications for experimental hepatopulmonary syndrome. Am J Physiol Lung Cell Mol Physiol 2007;292(6): L1467–72.
14. Schenk P, Madl C, Rezaie-Majd S, et al. Methylene blue improves the hepatopulmonary syndrome. Ann Intern Med 2000;133(9):701–6.
15. Nunes H, Lebrec D, Mazmanian M, et al. Role of nitric oxide in hepatopulmonary syndrome in cirrhotic rats. Am J Respir Crit Care Med 2001;164(5):879–85.
16. Rolla G, Brussino L, Colagrande P, et al. Exhaled nitric oxide and oxygenation abnormalities in hepatic cirrhosis. Hepatology 1997;26(4):842–7.
17. Cremona G, Higenbottam TW, Mayoral V, et al. Elevated exhaled nitric oxide in patients with hepatopulmonary syndrome. Eur Respir J 1995;8(11):1883–5.

18. Whyte MK, Hughes JM, Peters AM, et al. Analysis of intrapulmonary right to left shunt in the hepatopulmonary syndrome. J Hepatol 1998;29(1):85–93.
19. Edell ES, Cortese DA, Krowka MJ, et al. Severe hypoxemia and liver disease. Am Rev Respir Dis 1989;140(6):1631–5.
20. Martinez GP, Barbera JA, Visa J, et al. Hepatopulmonary syndrome in candidates for liver transplantation. J Hepatol 2001;34(5):651–7.
21. Rodriguez-Roisin R, Roca J, Agusti AG, et al. Gas exchange and pulmonary vascular reactivity in patients with liver cirrhosis. Am Rev Respir Dis 1987; 135(5):1085–92.
22. Krowka MJ, Wiseman GA, Burnett OL, et al. Hepatopulmonary syndrome: a prospective study of relationships between severity of liver disease, PaO(2) response to 100% oxygen, and brain uptake after (99m)Tc MAA lung scanning. Chest 2000;118(3):615–24.
23. Henriksen JH, Ring-Larsen H, Christensen NJ. Circulating noradrenaline and central haemodynamics in patients with cirrhosis. Scand J Gastroenterol 1985; 20(10):1185–90.
24. Thorens JB, Junod AF. Hypoxaemia and liver cirrhosis: a new argument in favour of a "diffusion-perfusion defect". Eur Respir J 1992;5(6):754–6.
25. Robin ED, Laman D, Horn BR, et al. Platypnea related to orthodeoxia caused by true vascular lung shunts. N Engl J Med 1976;294(17):941–3.
26. Gomez FP, Martinez-Palli G, Barbera JA, et al. Gas exchange mechanism of orthodeoxia in hepatopulmonary syndrome. Hepatology 2004;40(3):660–6.
27. Rodriguez-Roisin R, Krowka MJ, Herve P, et al. Pulmonary-hepatic vascular disorders (PHD). Eur Respir J 2004;24(5):861–80.
28. Krowka MJ, Dickson ER, Cortese DA. Hepatopulmonary syndrome. Clinical observations and lack of therapeutic response to somatostatin analogue. Chest 1993;104(2):515–21.
29. Martinez-Palli G, Gomez FP, Barbera JA, et al. Sustained low diffusing capacity in hepatopulmonary syndrome after liver transplantation. World J Gastroenterol 2006;12(36):5878–83.
30. Battaglia SE, Pretto JJ, Irving LB, et al. Resolution of gas exchange abnormalities and intrapulmonary shunting following liver transplantation. Hepatology 1997; 25(5):1228–32.
31. Abrams GA, Nanda NC, Dubovsky EV, et al. Use of macroaggregated albumin lung perfusion scan to diagnose hepatopulmonary syndrome: a new approach. Gastroenterology 1998;114(2):305–10.
32. Krowka MJ, Tajik AJ, Dickson ER, et al. Intrapulmonary vascular dilatations (IPVD) in liver transplant candidates. Screening by two-dimensional contrast-enhanced echocardiography. Chest 1990;97(5):1165–70.
33. Poterucha JJ, Krowka MJ, Dickson ER, et al. Failure of hepatopulmonary syndrome to resolve after liver transplantation and successful treatment with embolotherapy. Hepatology 1995;21(1):96–100.
34. Taille C, Cadranel J, Bellocq A, et al. Liver transplantation for hepatopulmonary syndrome: a ten-year experience in Paris, France. Transplantation 2003;75(9): 1482–9 [discussion: 1446–87].
35. Almeida JA, Riordan SM, Liu J, et al. Deleterious effect of nitric oxide inhibition in chronic hepatopulmonary syndrome. Eur J Gastroenterol Hepatol 2007;19(4): 341–6.
36. Mantz FA Jr, Craige E. Portal axis thrombosis with spontaneous portacaval shunt and resultant cor pulmonale. AMA Arch Pathol 1951;52(1):91–7.

37. Hoeper MM, Krowka MJ, Strassburg CP. Portopulmonary hypertension and hepatopulmonary syndrome. Lancet 2004;363(9419):1461–8.
38. Castro M, Krowka MJ, Schroeder DR, et al. Frequency and clinical implications of increased pulmonary artery pressures in liver transplant patients. Mayo Clin Proc 1996;71(6):543–51.
39. McDonnell PJ, Toye PA, Hutchins GM. Primary pulmonary hypertension and cirrhosis: are they related? Am Rev Respir Dis 1983;127(4):437–41.
40. Hadengue A, Benhayoun MK, Lebrec D, et al. Pulmonary hypertension complicating portal hypertension: prevalence and relation to splanchnic hemodynamics. Gastroenterology 1991;100(2):520–8.
41. Plevak D, Krowka M, Rettke S, et al. Successful liver transplantation in patients with mild to moderate pulmonary hypertension. Transplant Proc 1993;25(2):1840.
42. Benjaminov FS, Prentice M, Sniderman KW, et al. Portopulmonary hypertension in decompensated cirrhosis with refractory ascites. Gut 2003;52(9):1355–62.
43. Mandell MS, Groves BM. Pulmonary hypertension in chronic liver disease. Clin Chest Med 1996;17(1):17–33.
44. Panos RJ, Baker SK. Mediators, cytokines, and growth factors in liver-lung interactions. Clin Chest Med 1996;17(1):151–69.
45. Rockey DC. Vascular mediators in the injured liver. Hepatology 2003;37(1):4–12.
46. Robalino BD, Moodie DS. Association between primary pulmonary hypertension and portal hypertension: analysis of its pathophysiology and clinical, laboratory and hemodynamic manifestations. J Am Coll Cardiol 1991;17(2):492–8.
47. Krowka MJ, Porayko MK, Plevak DJ, et al. Hepatopulmonary syndrome with progressive hypoxemia as an indication for liver transplantation: case reports and literature review. Mayo Clin Proc 1997;72(1):44–53.
48. Edwards BS, Weir EK, Edwards WD, et al. Coexistent pulmonary and portal hypertension: morphologic and clinical features. J Am Coll Cardiol 1987;10(6):1233–8.
49. Krowka MJ. Hepatopulmonary syndrome versus portopulmonary hypertension: distinctions and dilemmas. Hepatology 1997;25(5):1282–4.
50. Torregrosa M, Genesca J, Gonzalez A, et al. Role of Doppler echocardiography in the assessment of portopulmonary hypertension in liver transplantation candidates. Transplantation 2001;71(4):572–4.
51. Krowka MJ. Pulmonary hypertension: diagnostics and therapeutics. Mayo Clin Proc 2000;75(6):625–30.
52. Shapiro SM, Oudiz RJ, Cao T, et al. Primary pulmonary hypertension: improved long-term effects and survival with continuous intravenous epoprostenol infusion. J Am Coll Cardiol 1997;30(2):343–9.
53. Barst RJ, Rubin LJ, Long WA, et al. A comparison of continuous intravenous epoprostenol (prostacyclin) with conventional therapy for primary pulmonary hypertension. The Primary Pulmonary Hypertension Study Group. N Engl J Med 1996;334(5):296–302.
54. Minder S, Fischler M, Muellhaupt B, et al. Intravenous iloprost bridging to orthotopic liver transplantation in portopulmonary hypertension. Eur Respir J 2004;24(4):703–7.
55. Halank M, Marx C, Miehlke S, et al. Use of aerosolized inhaled iloprost in the treatment of portopulmonary hypertension. J Gastroenterol 2004;39(12):1222–3.
56. Chua R, Keogh A, Miyashita M. Novel use of sildenafil in the treatment of portopulmonary hypertension. J Heart Lung Transplant 2005;24(4):498–500.

57. Krowka MJ, Mandell MS, Ramsay MA, et al. Hepatopulmonary syndrome and portopulmonary hypertension: a report of the multicenter liver transplant database. Liver Transpl 2004;10(2):174–82.
58. Swanson KL, Wiesner RH, Nyberg SL, et al. Survival in portopulmonary hypertension: mayo clinic experience categorized by treatment subgroups. Am J Transplant 2008;8(11):2445–53.
59. Kotloff RM, Ahya VN, Crawford SW. Pulmonary complications of solid organ and hematopoietic stem cell transplantation. Am J Respir Crit Care Med 2004;170(1): 22–48.
60. Kett DH, Acosta RC, Campos MA, et al. Recurrent portopulmonary hypertension after liver transplantation: management with epoprostenol and resolution after retransplantation. Liver Transpl 2001;7(7):645–8.
61. Kuo PC, Plotkin JS, Gaine S, et al. Portopulmonary hypertension and the liver transplant candidate. Transplantation 1999;67(8):1087–93.
62. Huang TW, Cheng YL, Chang H, et al. Education and imaging. Hepatobiliary and pancreatic: hepatic hydrothorax. J Gastroenterol Hepatol 2007;22(6):956.
63. Wilputte JY, Goffette P, Zech F, et al. The outcome after transjugular intrahepatic portosystemic shunt (TIPS) for hepatic hydrothorax is closely related to liver dysfunction: a long-term study in 28 patients. Acta Gastroenterol Belg 2007; 70(1):6–10.
64. Ibrisim D, Cakaloglu Y, Akyuz F, et al. Treatment of hepatic hydrothorax with terlipressin in a cirrhotic patient. Scand J Gastroenterol 2006;41(7):862–5.
65. Barreales M, Saenz-Lopez S, Igarzabal A, et al. Refractory hepatic hydrothorax: successful treatment with octreotide. Rev Esp Enferm Dig 2005;97(11):830–5.

Current Management of Hepatocellular Carcinoma

Manuel Mendizabal, MD[a], K. Rajender Reddy, MD[b],*

KEYWORDS

- Hepatocellular carcinoma • Liver
- Liver transplantation • Sorafenib

Hepatocellular carcinoma (HCC) is a major health problem and a leading cause of mortality among patients with cirrhosis. It is the sixth most common neoplasm worldwide and the third leading cause of death attributable to cancer.[1] In the United States the incidence of HCC has risen during the last few decades from 1.3 per 100,000 population between 1978 and 1980 to 3.3 per 100,000 population between 1998 and 2001.[2,3] This increasing incidence is likely to continue in the coming years, primarily because of progressive liver disease attributable to hepatitis C virus (HCV) in those individuals who became infected a few decades ago.[4] However, because hepatitis B virus (HBV) infection is more prevalent than HCV globally, HBV remains the single most important cause of HCC worldwide and particularly remains high in Asia and Africa relative to Western populations.

The annual incidence of HCC among patients with cirrhosis is between 2% and 6%.[2,5–7] HCC carries a poor prognosis and is rarely cured when diagnosed in a symptomatic stage. Several studies have shown that treatment is more effective when HCC is diagnosed at an early stage.[2,8,9] As part of active surveillance, more asymptomatic patients are being diagnosed. In addition, there are several treatments available that have a positive impact on survival.[10] Treatment of HCC is multidisciplinary and involves hepatologists, oncologists, surgeons, and interventional radiologists.

The purpose of this review is to examine the strategy for conducting HCC surveillance, diagnosing this malignancy, particularly at an early stage, and pursuing effective treatment options.

SURVEILLANCE

The objective of HCC surveillance is to reduce mortality from the disease. A large randomized controlled trial showed that HCC surveillance with liver ultrasound (US)

[a] Servicio de Hepatología, Trasplante Hepático y Cirugía Hepatobiliar, Hospital Universitario Austral, Pilar, Argentina
[b] Department of Medicine, University of Pennsylvania, 2 Dulles, HUP, 3400 Spruce Street, Philadelphia, PA 19104, USA
* Corresponding author.
E-mail address: rajender.reddy@uphs.upenn.edu (K.R. Reddy).

Med Clin N Am 93 (2009) 885–900
doi:10.1016/j.mcna.2009.03.004
0025-7125/09/$ – see front matter © 2009 Elsevier Inc. All rights reserved.

and serum α-fetoprotein (AFP) every 6 months improved survival.[11] HCC mortality was reduced by 37%, although adherence to surveillance was less than 60%. Surveillance should be offered to those patients who are at high risk of developing HCC (**Box 1**). Liver US and serum AFP are the most accepted tests for HCC surveillance. With regard to AFP, an optimal balance between sensitivity and specificity is achieved by a cutoff level of 20 ng/mL.[12] However, at this level the sensitivity is only 60%, and therefore it is considered inadequate as the sole screening test.[13,14] AFP still has a role in the diagnosis of HCC, because a level above 200 ng/mL in a patient with cirrhosis and with a liver mass is diagnostic for HCC.[12] The poor performance of total AFP in detecting HCC has led to increased interest in identifying other tumor markers that may have a greater clinical utility. Two new markers have received the most attention, des-γ-carboxyprothrombin (DCP) and lectin-bound AFP (AFP-L3), and both are routinely used in Japan. DCP has been found to have a direct correlation with tumor size,[15] whereas AFP-L3 was reported to be a more specific marker for HCC than AFP, and a combined use of both was described to be helpful in reducing the relatively high false-positive rate of total AFP alone.[16] It has also been suggested that a combination of these 3 markers could identify individuals with negative imaging results who would benefit from follow-up evaluation.[17] On the other hand, different studies exhibited great disparity of AFP-L3 sensitivity as a screening test for HCC, ranging between 30% and 96%.[18–20] Although these tumor markers present promising results, their routine use is not yet recommended.

The sensitivity of US is between 58% and 78%, and the specificity is greater than 90% when it is used as a surveillance test;[2] and this performance is superior to that of any of the serologic tests. However, sensitivity of US is particularly low to detect tumor nodules in cirrhotic livers.[21,22] In addition, US performance is operator-dependent and is technically more difficult in obese patients. Current guidelines, based on tumor growth rates, recommend US surveillance intervals of 6 to 12 months, and AFP alone should be used only if US is unavailable.[23]

Box 1
High-risk groups in whom HCC surveillance is recommended

Hepatitis B carriers

Asian males ≥ 40 years

Asian females ≥ 50 years

All cirrhotic HBV carriers

Family history of HCC

Africans > 20 years

Non-hepatitis B cirrhosis

Hepatitis C

Alcoholic cirrhosis

Genetic hemochromatosis

Primary biliary cirrhosis

No recommendations for or against surveillance

α-1 Antitrypsin deficiency

Nonalcoholic steatohepatitis

Autoimmune hepatitis

Combined use of US and AFP increases not only detection rates but also cost and false-positive rates.[24] CT scan and MRI are diagnostic tests and not meant for surveillance; their cost and associated radiation and contrast exposure do not make them cost-effective.

Once a solitary mass or multiple masses are detected on US surveillance in a patient with cirrhosis, it is important to demonstrate that they represent HCC and, eventually, the stage is determined. Triple-phase spiral CT and dynamic MRI are the diagnostic tests of choice.[25,26] The tumor has an exclusive blood supply from the hepatic artery that demonstrates contrast uptake during the early arterial phase and washout in the delay venous phase. Washout is defined as a hypointensity of a nodule in the delayed phases of MRI or CT examination compared with the surrounding liver.[27] It is thought to be caused by greater neovascularization in HCC tumors than in the surrounding hepatic parenchyma, presenting an early venous drainage in delayed images (**Fig. 1**). Arterial enhancement with washout of a mass in a cirrhotic liver has a sensitivity of 90% and a specificity of 95% for the diagnosis of cirrhosis.[28] Various studies have demonstrated that MRI is slightly better than CT in the characterization and diagnosis of HCC.[29–31] MRI and CT accuracy is affected by the tumor size; MRI has been described to have a rate of detection for HCC of greater than 95% in those lesions larger than 2 cm and only 33% for those smaller than 2 cm.[32]

DIAGNOSIS

Based on the growing availability of potential curative therapies that may improve survival in selected patients, the diagnosis of HCC is of considerable interest to

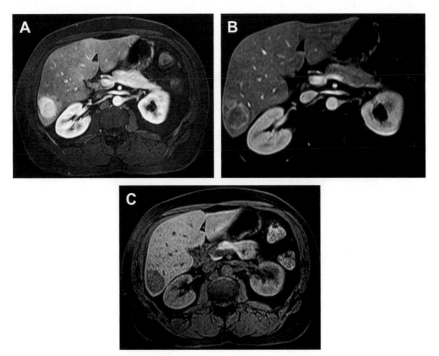

Fig. 1. Early arterial phase and washout in the delay venous phase of hepatic tumor. (*A*) arterial phase enhancement; (*B*) delayed washout; (*C*) early washout.

clinicians evaluating patients with liver cirrhosis. An algorithm for the evaluation of a patient with an abnormal surveillance test for HCC has been recommended[23] (**Fig. 2**). Diagnosis of HCC can be made in patients with cirrhosis who have a focal hepatic mass greater than 2 cm identified on one dynamic imaging technique with a typical vascular pattern (arterial enhancement with washout). In those patients with liver lesion greater than 2 cm but an atypical vascular pattern on imaging, a biopsy is recommended.

Focal hepatic lesions on screening of a cirrhotic liver between 1 and 2 cm presenting characteristic arterial enhancement features with venous washout on 2 different imaging modalities should be treated as HCC. On the other hand, if a typical vascular pattern is detected on only one imaging study, a biopsy should be considered. Finally, nodules smaller than 1 cm in diameter need to be followed up every 3 to 4 months to detect growth suggestive of malignant transformation. If the hepatic lesion remains stable after 2 years, it is suggested that the patients return to the standard surveillance protocol of every 6 to 12 months.[23,33]

STAGING

A precise staging of the tumor before considering treatment of HCC is helpful to estimate prognosis and decide as to which therapy may offer the greatest survival potential. Several prognostic staging systems have been proposed,[34–37] but the Barcelona-Clinic Liver Cancer (BCLC) staging system is the most widely accepted. The BCLC prognostic system accounts for different factors of performance status, tumor burden, and hepatic function and categorizes patients into 5 stages which then helps select the ideal candidates for the therapies currently available. The BCLC staging system is the only system that links tumor staging with treatment strategy (**Fig. 3**). This system has been recently validated by an external cohort study wherein the BCLC staging system offered better prognostic power than other staging systems.[38] The *very early* HCC includes patients presenting with a single lesion less than 2 cm who are asymptomatic and have no vascular invasion. In Child-Pugh class A, a survival of 90% and 71% after 5 years can be achieved with resection or radiofrequency ablation (RFA), respectively.[39,40] *Early-stage* disease is characterized by preserved liver function (Child-Pugh class A and B), a single HCC of 5 cm or less, or up to 3 lesions less than 3 cm in size. These patients can be treated effectively by orthotopic liver transplantation (OLT), resection, often if solitary, or percutaneous ablation with 5-year survival figures up to 75%. The *intermediate-stage* HCC corresponds to patients with large/multifocal HCC, without symptoms and no evident vascular invasion. These are optimal candidates for transarterial chemoembolization (TACE). Patients who have symptomatic tumors and/or invasive tumoral pattern (vascular invasion/extrahepatic spread) comprise the *advance stage*. This group of patients may benefit from new agents such as sorafenib, which has recently showed improved overall survival. Finally, *terminal stage* HCC represents those patients who have end-stage liver disease and extensive tumor burden, and they have extremely grim prognosis. Unfortunately, they are not likely to benefit with any of the treatments aforementioned and should only receive symptomatic treatment.

TREATMENT
Surgical Resection

Resection is the treatment of choice for noncirrhotic patients who have HCC; however, these patients account for only about 5% of patients in Western countries and for about 40% in Asian populations (except Japan).[2] Among patients who have cirrhosis,

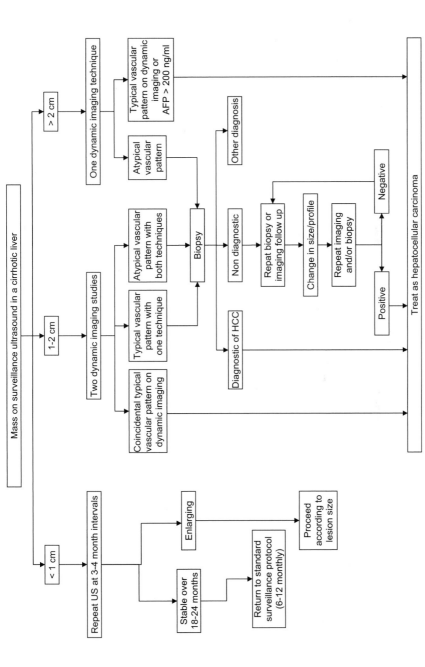

Fig. 2. Surveillance and diagnosis algorithm as recommended by the American Association for the Study of Liver Diseases guideline. US, ultrasound; AFP, alpha-fetoprotein. (*From* Bruix J, Sherman M. Management of hepatocellular carcinoma. Hepatology 2005;42:1217; with permission.)

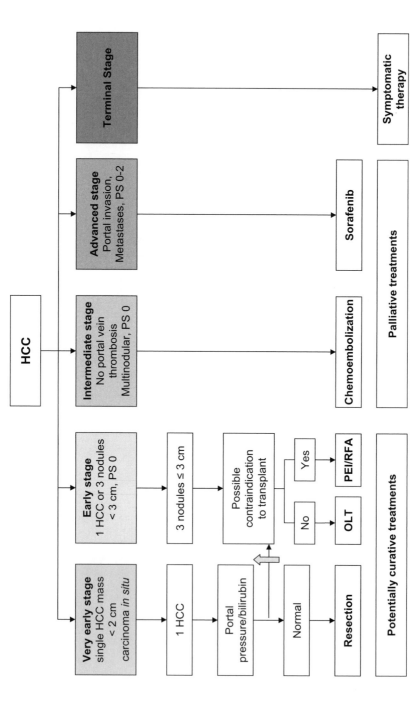

Fig. 3. A treatment strategy based on stage of tumor and performance characteristics. OLT, orthotopic liver transplantation; PEI, percutaneous ethanol injection; PS, performance status; RFA, radiofrequency ablation. (*From* El-Serag HB, Marrero JA, Rudolph L, et al. Diagnosis and treatment of hepato-cellular carcinoma. Gastroenterology 2008;134(6):1752; with permission.)

strict selection criteria are required to avoid hepatic decompensation. The selection of candidates is based on normal bilirubin level; absence of significant portal hypertension, defined as hepatic vein pressure gradient less than 10 mmHg; absence of varices; and platelet count higher than 100,000/mm³. Selected patients can achieve a survival rate higher than 70% at 5 years;[36] however, with application of these criteria the resectability rate is 5% to 10%. Tumor recurrence rates of 50% at 3 years and 70% at 5 years are seen after resection, and this is potentially likely from multiple factors that include the growth of occult neoplastic foci in the remnant liver, an inadequate resection margin, or an ongoing carcinogenic process associated with cirrhosis.[7,36,41–43] The risk of recurrence is affected by several variables including microvascular invasion, multinodularity, tumor size, and width of the tumor-free resection margin.[43–46] A single tumor of 5 cm or less is associated with a favorable outcome after liver resection because the risks of dissemination and vascular invasion decrease with such size of the tumor.[46] Thus far, only adjuvant interferon-α treatment has showed beneficial effects after hepatic resection,[47] especially in patients with HBV infection;[48,49] on the other hand, preoperative chemoembolization or chemotherapy are not effective.[50,51] Intraoperative US enables the detection of nodules between 0.5 and 1 cm, and is often used intraoperatively to identify any additional nodules and also guide anatomic resections.[10,52]

Liver Transplantation

In patients who are not candidates for hepatic resection because of one or more reasons of location, multicentricity, portal hypertension, inadequate functional hepatic reserve, and the risk of postoperative decompensation, OLT offers curative therapy, as well as amelioration of the underlying cirrhosis. The initial experiences of OLT for HCC were dismal in that 5-year recurrence and survival rates were 50% and less than 40%, respectively.[53–55] The landmark study of Mazzaferro and colleagues,[56] in 1996, noted that when OLT was restricted to patients with solitary HCC of 5 cm or less, or with up to 3 nodules, each smaller than 3 cm in diameter, the survival rate after 5 years exceeded 70%, with a low recurrence of less than 15%. These outcomes are comparable to those of OLT for patients who do not have HCC. The criteria developed by Mazzaferro and colleagues have come to be known as the Milan criteria and have been applied around the world, including by the United Network of Organ Sharing (UNOS), in the selection of patients with HCC for transplantation. Organ allocation policy is based on the Model for End-Stage Liver Disease (MELD) score, and patients with HCC are being awarded exception points to shorten their waiting time with a reasonable expectation of being transplanted in a time frame that would allow for tumor stability. The exception points for HCC are based on the expected 3-month pretransplantation mortality rates. Patients meeting the Milan criteria receive a MELD score of 22, equivalent to a 15% probability of death within 3 months, unless their calculated MELD score is otherwise greater. Every 3 months, for patients remaining on the waiting list and within Milan criteria, the MELD score is increased to account for an additional 10% increase in mortality risk.

The University of California in San Francisco (UCSF) has proposed that a modest expansion of tumor size beyond the Milan criteria (1 tumor ≤ 6.5 cm or up to 3 lesions each ≤ 4.5 cm with a total tumor diameter ≤ 8 cm) could achieve posttransplant survival comparable to that with the Milan criteria. These criteria were initially derived from tumor explant characteristics,[57] and it has been recently validated in a separate cohort at UCSF with selection criteria based on imaging studies.[58] The 1- and 5-year recurrence-free probabilities were 95% and 90%, and the respective survivals without recurrence were 92% and 80%. Although promising, these results should be confirmed by other centers before changing the current criteria. Further, the challenge is to keep a balance of organ allocation and transplantation, with successful and comparable outcomes between HCC and non-HCC advanced liver disease recipients.

An attractive strategy to improve the results of OLT for expanded criteria HCC is downstaging to within Milan criteria using locoregional therapy with one or more therapeutic modalities including percutaneous ethanol injection (PEI), TACE, or RFA. Several studies have reported that downstaging can be achieved in up to 70% of the patients treated with various modalities.[59–61] Subsequently, selected patients underwent successful OLT with tumor-free and overall survival outcomes comparable to those transplanted with conventional criteria.[61,62] Theoretically, the fundamental principle behind downstaging is to select a subset of tumors with more favorable biology that are more likely to respond to treatment and then do well after OLT.[63] Although encouraging, all these reports included small numbers of patients with different selection criteria, pretransplant treatment, and waiting time, and therefore a direct comparison is not possible. There is still a need for refinement of downstaging treatments and criteria for selection of candidates for OLT before such a strategy is recommended and adopted.

Liver transplantation for HCC is limited by the shortage of organs, with up to 30% of patients developing contraindications while waiting for a donor.[64,65] Living donor liver transplantation (LDLT) potentially can eliminate the significant waiting time and allow the surgery to be performed electively. LDLT is a complex intervention associated with 20% to 40% donor morbidity and 0.3% to 0.5% donor mortality.[66] Results from different studies from Asia suggest that the outcome for the recipient after LDLT is the same as with cadaveric donation.[67–69] On the other hand, a recent retrospective study from the United States found that patients with HCC who underwent LDLT had a significantly higher HCC recurrence rate than did their cadaveric liver transplantation counterparts.[70] However, the overall mortality and 3-year recurrence-free survival rates were similar in both groups. Thus, the role of LDLT in HCC recipients requires further evaluation. Recipient characteristics of tumor burden, age, and severity of underlying liver disease, in addition to donor criteria, such as degree of hepatic steatosis and age, may influence outcomes.

Percutaneous Ablation

Percutaneous ablation is the initial option for patients who are afflicted with early HCC and who are not candidates for resection or OLT. Ablation of tumor cells may be accomplished either by chemicals (eg, ethanol or acetic acid) or by physiologic techniques (eg, radiofrequency, microwave, or cryoablation). Although not entirely reliable, response is considered to have occurred when a CT or MRI evaluation shows an extensive nonenhancing low-density area, reflecting complete tumor necrosis.[7]

PEI was the first percutaneous technique introduced in clinical practice and is usually performed under US guidance. It has been reported to induce chemical coagulative necrosis in 70% to 80% of solitary HCC 3 cm or less and in almost 100% in tumors less than 2 cm; however, its efficacy drops to 50% in lesions between 3 and 5 cm.[71,72] It is a safe, inexpensive, and well-tolerated procedure but requires repeated injections on separated days. This procedure, however, carries a small but definite risk of needle track seeding and is not a desirable procedure in the context of liver transplantation.[73]

RFA achieves a similar level of response as PEI in tumors less than 2 cm but with fewer sessions and may produce better results in tumors greater than 2 cm.[74–77] During the past few years, 5 randomized clinical trials (RCTs) compared RFA with PEI in treating patients with small HCC less than 5 cm (**Table 1**). Three studies from

Table 1
Randomized clinical trials that compared percutaneous ethanol injection versus radiofrequency ablation in Child A/B patients

Author	N (PEI/RFA)	Tumor Size	Tumor Necrosis Rate PEI/RFA (%)	Survival Difference
Brunello and colleagues[79]	69/70	<3 lesions, <3 cm each	65/95	No
Lencioni and colleagues[74]	50/52	Milan criteria	82/91	No[a]
Shiina and colleagues[77]	114/118	<3 lesions, <3 cm each	NA	Yes
Lin and colleagues[75] (2004)	52/52	<3 lesions, ≤4 cm each	88/96	Yes
Lin and colleagues[78] (2005)	62/62	<3 lesions, ≤3 cm each	88/96	Yes

[a] RFA > PEI local recurrence free and events free.

Asia showed survival advantages favoring RFA over PEI.[75,77,78] Conversely, no differences in survival were reported in the 2 European RCTs.[74,79] Overall, RFA demonstrated superior efficacy in terms of lower local recurrence and longer disease-free survival. Local tumor control was reported to range between 91% and 96% for RFA and between 65% and 88% for PEI. It has been speculated that the injected ethanol cannot access the entire tumor volume due to intratumoral fibrotic septa. Both treatment groups presented similar adverse events; only one study found RFA to produce more major complications (4.8%).[78] Teratani and colleagues[80] reported that RFA can be performed effectively on nodules at high-risk locations (eg, close to large vessels and extrahepatic organs) by an experienced and skilled surgeon. On the other hand, subcapsular locations have been associated with increased risk of peritoneal seeding.[81] Nowadays, because of its better local tumor control and longer overall survival for patients with tumors less than 4 cm, RFA is the ablative procedure of choice in most centers.

After the introduction of percutaneous ablation techniques, their efficacy compared with resection in the treatment of small HCC has been debated. Two recent RCTs found no significant differences in overall survival and disease-free survival between resection and PEI or RFA.[82,83] A large Japanese prospective study that included 7185 patients with small HCC divided the patients into those undergoing hepatic resection versus RFA versus PEI.[84] The time-to-recurrence was significantly lower for the resection group; however, no difference was found in overall survival for all 3 groups. Another series recently published from the Surveillance, Epidemiology and End Results database[85] included patients with HCC within Milan criteria and compared overall survival for OLT, resection, and ablation. As expected, OLT had the best outcome, followed by resection and percutaneous ablation. Actuarial survival at 5 years was 43% after resection and 16% after ablation. The ablation group included different techniques (RFA, PEI, and cryosurgery).

Transarterial Chemoembolization

Patients who have compensated cirrhosis and HCC outside of the *early-stage* criteria and who do not have extrahepatic metastasis, vascular invasion, or cancer-related symptoms are included in the *intermediate stage*. TACE has been proven to be effective in this group.[86,87] The procedure consists of administration of an embolizing agent into the hepatic artery (transarterial embolization) with or without the injection of one or more chemotherapy drugs (TACE) and a contrast agent, lipiodol. At least 2 meta-analyses compared embolization and/or chemoembolization with conservative management.[86,87] The first one found a significant improvement in the 2-year survival with TACE (odds ratio, 0.53, 95% confidence interval, 0.32–0.89) but not for embolization alone.[87] The second study also showed significant survival benefit of TACE over the control group, but did not show a survival benefit of TACE over embolization alone.[86] Takayasu and colleagues[88] reported a large prospective cohort study including 8510 patients with unresectable HCC who were treated with TACE; the median survival rate was 34 months with an overall survival at 1, 3, 5, and 7 years of 82%, 47%, 26%, and 16%, respectively. There is no good evidence for the best chemotherapeutic agent and the optimal re-treatment strategy. The most widely used chemotherapeutic drug is doxorubicin (36%), followed by cisplatin (31%).[87] It is generally accepted that maximal tumor response is achieved after repeated interventions, usually between 3 and 4 courses.[86,87,89]

Careful selection of patients for TACE should be undertaken. The benefits of chemoembolization should not be offset by treatment-induced liver failure. The main contraindication is portal vein thrombosis. Patients with advanced liver dysfunction (Child-Pugh class B or C), renal failure, vascular invasion, or extrahepatic tumor spread should be excluded from these treatments because they have increased risk of liver failure and death. Side effects are well described in patients undergoing transarterial embolization/TACE, and these include nausea, vomiting, ischemic cholecystitis, alopecia, and bone marrow depression in approximately 10% of the cases.[90] More than 50% of the patients treated with TACE suffer from the postembolization syndrome that includes fever, abdominal pain, and ileus. The mortality rate is less than 5%.[88,90] Prophylactic antibiotics are not routinely used.[91]

In summary, TACE is generally pursued in 3 clinical scenarios: (1) patients at the *intermediate-stage* of HCC; (2) the downstaging of tumors that exceed criteria for transplantation, although this is investigational; and (3) patients in whom RFA cannot be performed because of technical difficulties (proximity to blood vessel, gallbladder, or biliary tree) or high risk of tumor seeding (close to liver capsule).

Systemic Treatment

HCC has a dismal prognosis when it is diagnosed at an advanced stage or with progression after locoregional therapy. Systemic chemotherapy and hormonal compounds for HCC have been ineffective, with low response rates and no demonstrated survival benefit.[92,93] Systemic doxorubicin has been evaluated in more than 1000 patients within clinical trials and has provided partial responses in 10% of cases, without any evidence of survival benefit.[92] A meta-analysis of 7 RCTs showed that tamoxifen, an antiestrogen, does not provide significant antitumoral effect or survival benefit.[86]

The introduction of molecular targeted therapies that attack pathways that are critical for cancer survival and progression has created a new hope against this intractable cancer. The molecular pathogenesis of HCC has demonstrated the importance of activation of growth signaling pathways, including multiple receptor tyrosine kinase pathways, and inactivation of key tumor-suppressor genes.[94,95] Positive results have been reported with the use of sorafenib, an oral multikinase inhibitor, which inhibits tumor-cell proliferation and tumor angiogenesis and increases the rate of apoptosis in a wide range of tumor models.[96] A randomized phase III double-blind placebo-controlled trial in 602 patients with advanced HCC, treated with sorafenib, has shown a 3-month survival improvement.[97] The median overall survival was 10.7 months with sorafenib and 7.9 months with placebo (*P*<.001). Median time to progression was 5.5 months with sorafenib versus 2.8 months with placebo (*P*<.001). These results have set a benchmark for the management of HCC at an *advanced stage* or an *intermediate stage* not suitable for TACE but in well compensated liver disease patients (Child-Pugh class A). Although this therapy is exciting, we need to address more questions, such as the safety and benefit in the context of liver transplantation, and the benefit in those with advanced liver disease, as adjunctive therapy and as part of a multimodality approach.

Several studies evaluating the efficacy of different molecular therapies in HCC, alone or in combination with classical chemotherapy, are underway. The excitement resulting from the survival benefits obtained with these drugs in patients with breast cancer (bevacizumab), lung cancer (erlotinib), and liver metastases (cetuximab) provides a hope for patients suffering from HCC. These drugs are being tested in clinical trials in patients with HCC.

SUMMARY

The number of patients with HCC will continue to increase over the next decade. The overall survival has improved minimally over the last 20 years. Early detection at a presymptomatic stage is crucial for a potentially curative therapy. Considerable advances have been made in the ability to diagnose HCC. However, new biomarkers to establish the risk of cancer in cirrhotic patients and reliably diagnose HCC are needed. Surgical modalities, particularly liver transplantation, offer the best chance of a cure. Sorafenib is the first systemic therapy to prolong survival in advanced HCC, representing a breakthrough in the management of this complex disease. Combination trials exploring the potential efficacy of sorafenib with other classes of molecular agents and/or chemotherapeutics should be assessed.

REFERENCES

1. Parkin DM, Bray F, Ferlay J, et al. Global cancer statistics, 2002. CA Cancer J Clin 2005;55(2):74–108.
2. Bolondi L, Sofia S, Siringo S, et al. Surveillance programme of cirrhotic patients for early diagnosis and treatment of hepatocellular carcinoma: a cost effectiveness analysis. Gut 2001;48(2):251–9.
3. El-Serag HB, Rudolph KL. Hepatocellular carcinoma: epidemiology and molecular carcinogenesis. Gastroenterology 2007;132(7):2557–76.
4. El-Serag HB, Davila JA, Petersen NJ, et al. The continuing increase in the incidence of hepatocellular carcinoma in the United States: an update. Ann Intern Med 2003;139(10):817–23.
5. Colombo M, de Franchis R, Del Ninno E, et al. Hepatocellular carcinoma in Italian patients with cirrhosis. N Engl J Med 1991;325(10):675–80.
6. Velazquez RF, Rodriguez M, Navascues CA, et al. Prospective analysis of risk factors for hepatocellular carcinoma in patients with liver cirrhosis. Hepatology 2003;37(3):520–7.
7. Bruix J, Sherman M, Llovet JM, et al. Clinical management of hepatocellular carcinoma. Conclusions of the Barcelona-2000 EASL conference. European Association for the Study of the Liver. J Hepatol 2001;35(3):421–30.
8. Oka H, Kurioka N, Kim K, et al. Prospective study of early detection of hepatocellular carcinoma in patients with cirrhosis. Hepatology 1990;12(4 Pt 1):680–7.
9. Wong LL, Limm WM, Severino R, et al. Improved survival with screening for hepatocellular carcinoma. Liver Transpl 2000;6(3):320–5.

10. Llovet JM, Bruix J. Novel advancements in the management of hepatocellular carcinoma in 2008. J Hepatol 2008;48(Suppl 1):S20–37.

11. Zhang BH, Yang BH, Tang ZY. Randomized controlled trial of screening for hepatocellular carcinoma. J Cancer Res Clin Oncol 2004;130(7):417–22.

12. Trevisani F, D'Intino PE, Morselli-Labate AM, et al. Serum alpha-fetoprotein for diagnosis of hepatocellular carcinoma in patients with chronic liver disease: influence of HBsAg and anti-HCV status. J Hepatol 2001;34(4):570–5.

13. Sherman M. Alphafetoprotein: an obituary. J Hepatol 2001;34(4):603–5.

14. Zoli M, Magalotti D, Bianchi G, et al. Efficacy of a surveillance program for early detection of hepatocellular carcinoma. Cancer 1996;78(5):977–85.

15. Durazo FA, Blatt LM, Corey WG, et al. Des-gamma-carboxyprothrombin, alpha-fetoprotein and AFP-L3 in patients with chronic hepatitis, cirrhosis and hepatocellular carcinoma. J Gastroenterol Hepatol 2008;23(10):1541–8.

16. Sterling RK, Jeffers L, Gordon F, et al. Clinical utility of AFP-L3% measurement in North American patients with HCV-related cirrhosis. Am J Gastroenterol 2007; 102(10):2196–205.

17. Sterling RK, Jeffers L, Gordon F, et al. Utility of Lens culinaris agglutinin-reactive fraction of alpha-fetoprotein and des-gamma-carboxy prothrombin, alone or in combination, as biomarkers for hepatocellular carcinoma. Clin Gastroenterol Hepatol 2009;7(1):104–13.

18. Oka H, Saito A, Ito K, et al. Multicenter prospective analysis of newly diagnosed hepatocellular carcinoma with respect to the percentage of lens culinaris agglutinin-reactive alpha-fetoprotein. J Gastroenterol Hepatol 2001;16(12):1378–83.

19. Taketa K, Endo Y, Sekiya C, et al. A collaborative study for the evaluation of lectin-reactive alpha-fetoproteins in early detection of hepatocellular carcinoma. Cancer Res 1993;53(22):5419–23.

20. Khien VV, Mao HV, Chinh TT, et al. Clinical evaluation of lentil lectin-reactive alpha-fetoprotein-L3 in histology-proven hepatocellular carcinoma. Int J Biol Markers 2001;16(2):105–11.

21. Chen TH, Chen CJ, Yen MF, et al. Ultrasound screening and risk factors for death from hepatocellular carcinoma in a high risk group in Taiwan. Int J Cancer 2002; 98(2):257–61.

22. Kim CK, Lim JH, Lee WJ. Detection of hepatocellular carcinomas and dysplastic nodules in cirrhotic liver: accuracy of ultrasonography in transplant patients. J Ultrasound Med 2001;20(2):99–104.

23. Bruix J, Sherman M. Management of hepatocellular carcinoma. Hepatology 2005; 42(5):1208–36.

24. Zhang B, Yang B. Combined alpha fetoprotein testing and ultrasonography as a screening test for primary liver cancer. J Med Screen 1999;6(2):108–10.

25. Arguedas MR, Chen VK, Eloubeidi MA, et al. Screening for hepatocellular carcinoma in patients with hepatitis C cirrhosis: a cost-utility analysis. Am J Gastroenterol 2003;98(3):679–90.

26. Choi D, Kim SH, Lim JH, et al. Detection of hepatocellular carcinoma: combined T2-weighted and dynamic gadolinium-enhanced MRI versus combined CT during arterial portography and CT hepatic arteriography. J Comput Assist Tomogr 2001;25(5):777–85.

27. Hayashi M, Matsui O, Ueda K, et al. Progression to hypervascular hepatocellular carcinoma: correlation with intranodular blood supply evaluated with CT during intraarterial injection of contrast material. Radiology 2002;225(1):143–9.

28. El-Serag HB, Marrero JA, Rudolph L, et al. Diagnosis and treatment of hepatocellular carcinoma. Gastroenterology 2008;134(6):1752–63.

29. Burrel M, Llovet JM, Ayuso C, et al. MRI angiography is superior to helical CT for detection of HCC prior to liver transplantation: an explant correlation. Hepatology 2003;38(4):1034–42.
30. Libbrecht L, Bielen D, Verslype C, et al. Focal lesions in cirrhotic explant livers: pathological evaluation and accuracy of pretransplantation imaging examinations. Liver Transpl 2002;8(9):749–61.
31. Rode A, Bancel B, Douek P, et al. Small nodule detection in cirrhotic livers: evaluation with US, spiral CT, and MRI and correlation with pathologic examination of explanted liver. J Comput Assist Tomogr 2001;25(3): 327–36.
32. Ebara M, Ohto M, Watanabe Y, et al. Diagnosis of small hepatocellular carcinoma: correlation of MR imaging and tumor histologic studies. Radiology 1986;159(2): 371–7.
33. Byrnes V, Shi H, Kiryu S, et al. The clinical outcome of small (<20 mm) arterially enhancing nodules on MRI in the cirrhotic liver. Am J Gastroenterol 2007;102(8): 1654–9.
34. A new prognostic system for hepatocellular carcinoma: a retrospective study of 435 patients: the Cancer of the Liver Italian Program (CLIP) Investigators. Hepatology 1998;28(3):751–5.
35. Kudo M, Chung H, Osaki Y. Prognostic staging system for hepatocellular carcinoma (CLIP score): its value and limitations, and a proposal for a new staging system, the Japan integrated staging score (JIS score). J Gastroenterol 2003; 38(3):207–15.
36. Llovet JM, Bru C, Bruix J. Prognosis of hepatocellular carcinoma: the BCLC staging classification. Semin Liver Dis 1999;19(3):329–38.
37. Okuda K, Ohtsuki T, Obata H, et al. Natural history of hepatocellular carcinoma and prognosis in relation to treatment. Study of 850 patients. Cancer 1985; 56(4):918–28.
38. Marrero JA, Fontana RJ, Barrat A, et al. Prognosis of hepatocellular carcinoma: comparison of 7 staging systems in an American cohort. Hepatology 2005; 41(4):707–16.
39. Sakamoto M, Hirohashi S. Natural history and prognosis of adenomatous hyperplasia and early hepatocellular carcinoma: multi-institutional analysis of 53 nodules followed up for more than 6 months and 141 patients with single early hepatocellular carcinoma treated by surgical resection or percutaneous ethanol injection. Jpn J Clin Oncol 1998;28(10):604–8.
40. Takayama T, Makuuchi M, Hirohashi S, et al. Early hepatocellular carcinoma as an entity with a high rate of surgical cure. Hepatology 1998;28(5): 1241–6.
41. Imamura H, Matsuyama Y, Tanaka E, et al. Risk factors contributing to early and late phase intrahepatic recurrence of hepatocellular carcinoma after hepatectomy. J Hepatol 2003;38(2):200–7.
42. Okada S, Shimada K, Yamamoto J, et al. Predictive factors for postoperative recurrence of hepatocellular carcinoma. Gastroenterology 1994;106(6): 1618–24.
43. Poon RT, Fan ST, Lo CM, et al. Intrahepatic recurrence after curative resection of hepatocellular carcinoma: long-term results of treatment and prognostic factors. Ann Surg 1999;229(2):216–22.
44. Ikai I, Arii S, Kojiro M, et al. Reevaluation of prognostic factors for survival after liver resection in patients with hepatocellular carcinoma in a Japanese nationwide survey. Cancer 2004;101(4):796–802.

45. Llovet JM, Fuster J, Bruix J. Intention-to-treat analysis of surgical treatment for early hepatocellular carcinoma: resection versus transplantation. Hepatology 1999;30(6):1434–40.
46. Vauthey JN, Lauwers GY, Esnaola NF, et al. Simplified staging for hepatocellular carcinoma. J Clin Oncol 2002;20(6):1527–36.
47. Mazzaferro V, Romito R, Schiavo M, et al. Prevention of hepatocellular carcinoma recurrence with alpha-interferon after liver resection in HCV cirrhosis. Hepatology 2006;44(6):1543–54.
48. Sun HC, Tang ZY, Wang L, et al. Postoperative interferon alpha treatment postponed recurrence and improved overall survival in patients after curative resection of HBV-related hepatocellular carcinoma: a randomized clinical trial. J Cancer Res Clin Oncol 2006;132(7):458–65.
49. Lo CM, Liu CL, Chan SC, et al. A randomized, controlled trial of postoperative adjuvant interferon therapy after resection of hepatocellular carcinoma. Ann Surg 2007;245(6):831–42.
50. Schwartz JD, Schwartz M, Mandeli J, et al. Neoadjuvant and adjuvant therapy for resectable hepatocellular carcinoma: review of the randomised clinical trials. Lancet Oncol 2002;3(10):593–603.
51. Yamasaki S, Hasegawa H, Kinoshita H, et al. A prospective randomized trial of the preventive effect of pre-operative transcatheter arterial embolization against recurrence of hepatocellular carcinoma. Jpn J Cancer Res 1996; 87(2):206–11.
52. Torzilli G, Olivari N, Moroni E, et al. Contrast-enhanced intraoperative ultrasonography in surgery for hepatocellular carcinoma in cirrhosis. Liver Transpl 2004; 10(2 Suppl 1):S34–8.
53. Ringe B, Pichlmayr R, Wittekind C, et al. Surgical treatment of hepatocellular carcinoma: experience with liver resection and transplantation in 198 patients. World J Surg 1991;15(2):270–85.
54. Bismuth H, Chiche L, Adam R, et al. Liver resection versus transplantation for hepatocellular carcinoma in cirrhotic patients. Ann Surg 1993;218(2): 145–51.
55. Moreno P, Jaurrieta E, Figueras J, et al. Orthotopic liver transplantation: treatment of choice in cirrhotic patients with hepatocellular carcinoma? Transplant Proc 1995;27(4):2296–8.
56. Mazzaferro V, Regalia E, Doci R, et al. Liver transplantation for the treatment of small hepatocellular carcinomas in patients with cirrhosis. N Engl J Med 1996; 334(11):693–9.
57. Yao FY, Ferrell L, Bass NM, et al. Liver transplantation for hepatocellular carcinoma: expansion of the tumor size limits does not adversely impact survival. Hepatology 2001;33(6):1394–403.
58. Yao FY, Xiao L, Bass NM, et al. Liver transplantation for hepatocellular carcinoma: validation of the UCSF-expanded criteria based on preoperative imaging. Am J Transplant 2007;7(11):2587–96.
59. Yao FY. Liver transplantation for hepatocellular carcinoma: beyond the Milan criteria. Am J Transplant 2008;8(10):1982–9.
60. Yao FY, Hirose R, LaBerge JM, et al. A prospective study on downstaging of hepatocellular carcinoma prior to liver transplantation. Liver Transpl 2005; 11(12):1505–14.
61. Ravaioli M, Grazi GL, Piscaglia F, et al. Liver transplantation for hepatocellular carcinoma: results of down-staging in patients initially outside the Milan selection criteria. Am J Transplant 2008;8(12):2547–57.

62. Yao FY, Kerlan RK Jr, Hirose R, et al. Excellent outcome following down-staging of hepatocellular carcinoma prior to liver transplantation: an intention-to-treat analysis. Hepatology 2008;48(3):819–27.
63. Yao FY. Expanded criteria for hepatocellular carcinoma: down-staging with a view to liver transplantation–yes. Semin Liver Dis 2006;26(3):239–47.
64. Graziadei IW, Sandmueller H, Waldenberger P, et al. Chemoembolization followed by liver transplantation for hepatocellular carcinoma impedes tumor progression while on the waiting list and leads to excellent outcome. Liver Transpl 2003;9(6):557–63.
65. Yao FY, Bass NM, Nikolai B, et al. Liver transplantation for hepatocellular carcinoma: analysis of survival according to the intention-to-treat principle and dropout from the waiting list. Liver Transpl 2002;8(10):873–83.
66. Trotter JF, Wachs M, Everson GT, et al. Adult-to-adult transplantation of the right hepatic lobe from a living donor. N Engl J Med 2002;346(14): 1074–82.
67. Gondolesi GE, Roayaie S, Munoz L, et al. Adult living donor liver transplantation for patients with hepatocellular carcinoma: extending UNOS priority criteria. Ann Surg 2004;239(2):142–9.
68. Kaihara S, Kiuchi T, Ueda M, et al. Living-donor liver transplantation for hepatocellular carcinoma. Transplantation 2003;75(3 Suppl):S37–40.
69. Todo S, Furukawa H. Living donor liver transplantation for adult patients with hepatocellular carcinoma: experience in Japan. Ann Surg 2004;240(3):451–9 [discussion: 459–61].
70. Fisher RA, Kulik LM, Freise CE, et al. Hepatocellular carcinoma recurrence and death following living and deceased donor liver transplantation. Am J Transplant 2007;7(6):1601–8.
71. Ishii H, Okada S, Nose H, et al. Local recurrence of hepatocellular carcinoma after percutaneous ethanol injection. Cancer 1996;77(9):1792–6.
72. Livraghi T, Giorgio A, Marin G, et al. Hepatocellular carcinoma and cirrhosis in 746 patients: long-term results of percutaneous ethanol injection. Radiology 1995;197(1):101–8.
73. Ebara M, Okabe S, Kita K, et al. Percutaneous ethanol injection for small hepatocellular carcinoma: therapeutic efficacy based on 20-year observation. J Hepatol 2005;43(3):458–64.
74. Lencioni RA, Allgaier HP, Cioni D, et al. Small hepatocellular carcinoma in cirrhosis: randomized comparison of radio-frequency thermal ablation versus percutaneous ethanol injection. Radiology 2003;228(1):235–40.
75. Lin SM, Lin CJ, Lin CC, et al. Radiofrequency ablation improves prognosis compared with ethanol injection for hepatocellular carcinoma ≤4 cm. Gastroenterology 2004;127(6):1714–23.
76. Livraghi T, Goldberg SN, Lazzaroni S, et al. Small hepatocellular carcinoma: treatment with radio-frequency ablation versus ethanol injection. Radiology 1999; 210(3):655–61.
77. Shiina S, Teratani T, Obi S, et al. A randomized controlled trial of radiofrequency ablation with ethanol injection for small hepatocellular carcinoma. Gastroenterology 2005;129(1):122–30.
78. Lin SM, Lin CJ, Lin CC, et al. Randomised controlled trial comparing percutaneous radiofrequency thermal ablation, percutaneous ethanol injection, and percutaneous acetic acid injection to treat hepatocellular carcinoma of 3 cm or less. Gut 2005;54(8):1151–6.

79. Brunello F, Veltri A, Carucci P, et al. Radiofrequency ablation versus ethanol injection for early hepatocellular carcinoma: a randomized controlled trial. Scand J Gastroenterol 2008;43(6):727–35.

80. Teratani T, Yoshida H, Shiina S, et al. Radiofrequency ablation for hepatocellular carcinoma in so-called high-risk locations. Hepatology 2006;43(5):1101–8.

81. Llovet JM, Vilana R, Bru C, et al. Increased risk of tumor seeding after percutaneous radiofrequency ablation for single hepatocellular carcinoma. Hepatology 2001;33(5):1124–9.

82. Chen MS, Li JQ, Zheng Y, et al. A prospective randomized trial comparing percutaneous local ablative therapy and partial hepatectomy for small hepatocellular carcinoma. Ann Surg 2006;243(3):321–8.

83. Huang GT, Lee PH, Tsang YM, et al. Percutaneous ethanol injection versus surgical resection for the treatment of small hepatocellular carcinoma: a prospective study. Ann Surg 2005;242(1):36–42.

84. Hasegawa K, Makuuchi M, Takayama T, et al. Surgical resection vs percutaneous ablation for hepatocellular carcinoma: a preliminary report of the Japanese nationwide survey. J Hepatol 2008;49(4):589–94.

85. Schwarz RE, Smith DD. Trends in local therapy for hepatocellular carcinoma and survival outcomes in the US population. Am J Surg 2008;195(6):829–36.

86. Llovet JM, Bruix J. Systematic review of randomized trials for unresectable hepatocellular carcinoma: chemoembolization improves survival. Hepatology 2003; 37(2):429–42.

87. Marelli L, Stigliano R, Triantos C, et al. Transarterial therapy for hepatocellular carcinoma: which technique is more effective? A systematic review of cohort and randomized studies. Cardiovasc Intervent Radiol 2007;30(1):6–25.

88. Takayasu K, Arii S, Ikai I, et al. Prospective cohort study of transarterial chemoembolization for unresectable hepatocellular carcinoma in 8510 patients. Gastroenterology 2006;131(2):461–9.

89. Jaeger HJ, Mehring UM, Castaneda F, et al. Sequential transarterial chemoembolization for unresectable advanced hepatocellular carcinoma. Cardiovasc Intervent Radiol 1996;19(6):388–96.

90. Molinari M, Kachura JR, Dixon E, et al. Transarterial chemoembolisation for advanced hepatocellular carcinoma: results from a North American Cancer Centre. Clin Oncol (R Coll Radiol) 2006;18(9):684–92.

91. Castells A, Bruix J, Ayuso C, et al. Transarterial embolization for hepatocellular carcinoma. Antibiotic prophylaxis and clinical meaning of postembolization fever. J Hepatol 1995;22(4):410–5.

92. Lopez PM, Villanueva A, Llovet JM. Systematic review: evidence-based management of hepatocellular carcinoma–an updated analysis of randomized controlled trials. Aliment Pharmacol Ther 2006;23(11):1535–47.

93. Zhu AX. Systemic therapy of advanced hepatocellular carcinoma: how hopeful should we be? Oncologist 2006;11(7):790–800.

94. Llovet JM, Bruix J. Molecular targeted therapies in hepatocellular carcinoma. Hepatology 2008;48(4):1312–27.

95. Roberts LR. Sorafenib in liver cancer—just the beginning. N Engl J Med 2008; 359(4):420–2.

96. Chang YS, Adnane J, Trail PA, et al. Sorafenib (BAY 43-9006) inhibits tumor growth and vascularization and induces tumor apoptosis and hypoxia in RCC xenograft models. Cancer Chemother Pharmacol 2007;59(5):561–74.

97. Llovet JM, Ricci S, Mazzaferro V, et al. Sorafenib in advanced hepatocellular carcinoma. N Engl J Med 2008;359(4):378–90.

Health Maintenance Issues in Cirrhosis

Gaurav Mehta, MD, Kenneth D. Rothstein, MD*

KEYWORDS

• Cirrhosis • Vaccination • Abstinence • Nutrition • Analgesia

---

Liver cirrhosis is a relatively frequent cause of death in the United States accounting for more than 27,000 deaths every year.[1] Patients with liver cirrhosis have frequent medical complications and more so when the liver disease is more advanced and decompensated.[2] Patients with cirrhosis are considered to be immunocompromised. Some studies have suggested that the cost of managing liver disease may account for almost 1% of all healthcare spending.[3] All patients, especially those with cirrhosis, should have preventative measures and regular health maintenance. Patients should have regular medical checkups including screening for malignancy, osteoporosis, and routine vaccinations. Counseling for alcohol and tobacco abstinence should be emphasized at every visit. Special care should be given to prevent malnutrition in patients with advanced liver disease as the disease progresses. All patients with cirrhosis should maintain a healthy lifestyle in order to be candidates for liver transplantation should they eventually decompensate. This would include regular exercise, especially aerobic, and adherence to a healthy diet to keep their body mass index (BMI) close to normal. Patients with cirrhosis are at increased risk for both morbidity and mortality when they undergo surgery. The hepatologist's role should be to assist the primary care physician in maintaining the health of patients with cirrhosis. Specific recommendations should be discussed with each patient to optimize their health.

VACCINATIONS

More than 10,000 cases of acute hepatitis A were reported in the United States in 2001.[4] Periodic community epidemics have gradually decreased, probably because of better hygiene, improved water supplies, augmented food safety, and vaccination. The overall case-fatality ratio among cases reported through the National Notifiable Diseases Surveillance System is approximately 0.3% to 0.6% but reaches 1.8% among adults older than 50 years. Persons with chronic liver disease are at increased risk for acute liver failure.[5] Two serologic tests are licensed for the detection of antibodies to the hepatitis A virus (HAV): (1) IgM anti-HAV and (2) total anti-HAV (ie, IgM

Division of Gastroenterology and Hepatology, Department of Medicine, Drexel University College of Medicine, Mail Stop 913, 5th Floor, 219 N. Broad Street, Philadelphia, PA 19107, USA
* Corresponding author.
E-mail address: kenneth.rothstein@drexelmed.edu (K.D. Rothstein).

Med Clin N Am 93 (2009) 901–915
doi:10.1016/j.mcna.2009.03.005
0025-7125/09/$ – see front matter © 2009 Elsevier Inc. All rights reserved.

and IgG anti-HAV).[6] IgG anti-HAV, which appears early in the course of infection, remains detectable for a lifetime and provides lifelong protection against the disease. Although not at increased risk for the acquisition of HAV, persons with chronic liver disease are at an increased risk for fulminant hepatitis A.[7] Death certificate data indicate a higher prevalence of chronic liver disease among persons who died of fulminant hepatitis A when compared with persons who died of other causes.[5] Hence, all patients with cirrhosis should be screened and vaccinated for hepatitis A if they do not have IgG anti-HAV. Two formalin-inactivated hepatitis A virus vaccines were licensed by the Food and Drug Administration (FDA) for use in persons from 2 years of age and older. It should be given in 2 doses, at 0 and 6 months. The vaccine is slightly less immunogenic in patients with chronic liver disease (seroconversion rate, 93%).[8] The response to the vaccine should be checked with an IgG anti-HAV 3 months after the completion of the series. There is currently no consensus about nonresponders. Possible options include revaccination with either the standard dose or a double dose of the vaccine. Immune globulin can be given for passive immunoprophylaxis after exposure to hepatitis A or as pre-exposure prophylaxis in persons planning to travel to developing countries. It should ideally be given within 14 days after exposure.

In 2006, 4,758 cases of acute hepatitis B in the United States were reported to the Centers for Disease Control and Prevention (CDC). The overall incidence of reported acute hepatitis B was 1.6 in every 100,000 population, the lowest ever recorded. However, because many hepatitis B virus (HBV) infections are either asymptomatic or never reported, the actual number of new infections is estimated to be approximately tenfold higher. In 2006, an estimated 46,000 persons in the United States were newly infected with HBV.[9] The CDC has clearly stated in its guidelines that persons with chronic liver disease should get vaccinated for HBV.[10] This is performed not only to prevent hepatitis B infection but also to avoid the risk for decompensation in patients with advanced liver disease if they acquire acute hepatitis B. The vaccine is generally administered in 3 doses, with the second dose given 1 month after the first dose and the third dose given 6 months after the first dose. The antibody response declines with increasing age and in immunodeficiency states such as in patients with cirrhosis. Ideally, the antibody response is determined within 2 to 3 months after the last dose of the vaccine by measurement of anti-HBs antibody response. For persons who remain seronegative, a second series will result in seroconversion in 50% to 60% of recipients. For some patients a higher dose of 40 μg may be needed.[11] Hepatitis B immune globulin can be used to prevent hepatitis B infection in patients with cirrhosis without immunity to HBV who have been exposed to the virus after needle stick or sexual exposure.[12]

There is a vaccine available which combines the vaccines for hepatitis A and B called Twinrix. It is licensed for use in persons 18 years of age or older for whom both vaccines are indicated.[13] Immunization with Twinrix consists of 3 doses, given on a 0-, 1-, and 6-month schedule. Each 1-mL dose contains 720 ELISA units of inactivated hepatitis A virus and 20 mcg of hepatitis B surface antigen.

Patients with liver cirrhosis have impaired immunity and are susceptible to various communicable diseases. Patients with cirrhosis should have preventive measures similar to patients with other chronic conditions like renal failure and diabetes. Patients with cirrhosis with portosystemic shunting may have decreased clearance of bacteria, which may increase the severity of infection. Many of these patients have leukopenia, chemotactic defects, impaired cell-mediated immunity, and decreased complement activity. However, they are not considered immunosuppressed for the purpose of vaccination and are able to receive routine vaccinations with both inactivated and live vaccines according to the CDC guidelines.

Every year in the United States, 5% to 20% of the population gets the influenza virus. More than 200,000 people are hospitalized for flu complications and about 36,000 people die.[14] Patients with cirrhosis are at high risk for serious influenza complications. CDC recommends that patients with cirrhosis should be given yearly influenza vaccination as soon as the flu season begins in September. Most adults have antibody protection against influenza-virus infection within 2 weeks after vaccination.[15] There are 2 types of vaccines available for influenza. An inactivated vaccine (containing killed virus) that is given with a needle and a nasal-spray flu vaccine made with live, weakened flu viruses that do not cause the flu. The live vaccine is usually contraindicated for patients with altered immunocompetence and is indicated only for healthy individuals between the ages of 2 and 49 years. The CDC has no guidelines about using the live influenza vaccine in patients with cirrhosis. Flu vaccines will not protect against flu-like illnesses caused by noninfluenza viruses.

There are an estimated 175,000 hospitalized cases of pneumococcal pneumonia in the United States every year.[16] It is a common bacterial complication of influenza and measles. Pneumococcal disease is a leading cause of serious illness in children and adults throughout the world. The disease is caused by a common bacterium, the *Pneumococcus*, which can attack different parts of the body causing community-acquired bacterial pneumonia, bacteremia, and meningitis. The CDC recommends that patients with cirrhosis should get vaccinated once for *Pneumococcus*.

The CDC recommends that patients with cirrhosis should also be given an injection of the tetanus-diphtheria (Td) vaccine. This should be repeated every 10 years.

SCREENING FOR OSTEOPOROSIS

Osteoporosis is a major complication of chronic liver disease.[17] It can cause traumatic or spontaneous fractures, which can result in significant morbidity, decreased quality of life, and, in certain cases, reduced survival. Most fractures occur in the posttransplant setting but pretransplant osteoporosis is the main risk factor for posttransplant fractures. Although it is seen very well in chronic cholestatic conditions, osteoporosis occurs in cirrhosis from all etiologies, especially hepatitis C.[18] In end-stage primary biliary cirrhosis, the overall incidence of osteoporosis is around 40%, and fractures occur in about 21% of patients.[19] Several studies confirm a high rate of osteoporosis and osteopenia in patients with end-stage liver disease of varying etiologies. These studies have shown a variable incidence of osteoporosis (11%–48%) and osteopenia (18%–35%).[20–22]

There are multiple mechanisms and factors causing hepatic osteodystrophy in patients with advanced liver disease. Markers of bone formation are reduced in both cholestatic and noncholestatic liver disease. Unconjugated bilirubin impairs osteoblast proliferation.[23] Insulin-like growth factor 1, which is reduced in patients with cirrhosis, plays an important role in bone remodeling and maintenance of bone mass.[24] Sex hormone levels are important for regulation of bone mass. Hypogonadism is common in patients with advanced liver disease both in males and females. Hypogonadism results in increased-turnover bone loss and osteopenia.[20] Medications used in the treatment of liver diseases, such as corticosteroids, budesonide, and even interferon alfa, have reduced bone turnover and will inhibit the formation of osteoblasts.[25,26] Bile acid–binding agents such as cholestyramine can cause a decrease in absorption of vitamin D and 25-hydroxyvitamin D. Loop diuretics promote renal calcium loss, another source of decreased calcium in patients with cirrhosis.[27]

Osteoporosis is defined as a bone mass density of less than 2.5 standard deviations below normal adult peak bone mass, adjusted for male or female sex (T-score <-2.5). Osteopenia is a lesser degree of bone loss (T-score of -1.0 to -2.5). All patients with cirrhosis should be screened for osteoporosis. If the initial bone scan is normal, then repeat bone scans should be done every 3 to 5 years. If osteoporosis is detected on screening then specific therapy should be given followed by serial measurements of bone density. Therapy for osteoporosis includes biphosphonates[28]; calcitonin by subcutaneous or intranasal route, which has a relatively weak antiresorptive activity[29]; and hormone replacement therapy with the use of selective estrogen receptor modulators such as raloxifene.[30] Patients with osteopenia should also undergo serial bone scanning every 2 to 3 years. Supplementing with a calcium dose of 1500 mg/d for patients with cirrhosis who are at risk for osteopenia helps achieve positive calcium balance.[31] In a small study, supplementing with vitamin D showed benefits in patients with alcoholic cirrhosis.[32] The normal dose is about 50,000 IU of vitamin D orally 3 times a week. Regular exercise and adequate intake of proteins and calories can increase the mineral content of bones.

Testosterone levels of patients with cirrhosis should be checked as replacement promotes bone density and increases muscle mass. A level below 300 ng/dL is generally considered the threshold to start treatment, especially if there are symptoms. Treatment is available by means of an intramuscular injection every week, transdermal patches, or oral pills. After starting treatment, testosterone levels should be reassessed at 3 months and then yearly.

NUTRITIONAL ASPECTS IN CIRRHOSIS

The liver has a major role in the synthesis of plasma proteins, albumin, coagulation factors, lipoproteins, ketone bodies, and glucose to maintain glucose homeostasis. It accounts for about 20% of the body's resting energy requirements. Cirrhosis impairs hepatic function and causes decreased glucose, protein, and lipid metabolism.[33] Protein calorie malnutrition (PCM) is common in advanced liver disease with weight loss, nausea, and anorexia. About 20% of patients with Child-Pugh A cirrhosis and 60% with Child-Pugh C cirrhosis have PCM.[34]

The pathogenesis for malnutrition in cirrhosis is multifactorial. Patients with cirrhosis may have decreased food intake. There are several mechanisms that contribute to decreased food intake, which include decreased sweet, salty, and sour sensations. Early satiety associated with ascites,[35] dysgeusia because of vitamin A and zinc deficiency,[36] medication-induced nausea or anorexia, and psychological impairment alter eating behavior.[37] Malabsorption, caused by chronic cholestasis and decreased bile-salt-acid secretion, causes decreased fat and fat-soluble vitamin absorption.[38] Lactulose therapy can cause steatorrhea. Patients have impaired small-bowel motility and prolonged transit time,[39] which cause small-bowel bacterial overgrowth and malabsorption. Patients with alcoholic cirrhosis can have pancreatic insufficiency and cause further decrease in fat digestion and malabsorption. Patients with cirrhosis have a greater metabolic response to short-term starvation, causing a greater decline in hepatic glucose production, probably because of decreased hepatic glycogen and increased lipolysis of adipose tissue triglycerides.[40] Supplementing nocturnal nutrition in patients with cirrhosis has improved nutritional status and has increased body protein accretion. Skeletal muscle protein breakdown is often accelerated, which causes muscle wasting in patients with cirrhosis.[41]

PCM is associated with an increased risk for infections, esophageal variceal bleeding, and both renal and pulmonary complications. There is increased mortality after liver transplantation with increased risk for infections and prolonged hospitalization.[42] Muscle wasting found in patients with alcoholic cirrhosis is associated with increased postoperative mortality.[43] Several trials have shown that patients with alcoholic cirrhosis benefit from oral and enteral tube feedings. The patients have decreased hepatic encephalopathy, improvement in hepatic function, decreased Child-Pugh classification, and also improvement in overall survival.[44] Most patients can tolerate an increasing amount of protein without worsening encephalopathy. There should be no protein restriction as requirements are actually increased when there is cirrhosis. Encephalopathy should be managed with medications before protein restriction is instituted. Vegetable protein–based diets are preferred because they do not lead to encephalopathy.[45] Aggressive nutritional support is especially needed for patients awaiting transplantation to prevent wound dehiscence, infection, and, in severely malnourished patients, death after transplantation.[42] Patients should be monitored for hypoglycemia due to impaired gluconeogenesis, and they may require continuous dextrose infusion. Patients who are unable to meet the daily requirements may need enteral supplements. Nasoenteric feeds can be given safely even in patients with varices,[46] although they may be at a greater risk for aspiration and sinusitis. Percutaneous gastrostomy tubes should not be placed in patients with ascites, because this would cause leaking around the feeding tube and could cause an increased risk for infection.

Obesity has become a common problem in the United States. Obesity, hyperglycemia, type 2 diabetes, hypertriglyceridemia, and metabolic syndrome are the best known risk factors for nonalcoholic steatohepatitis (NASH).[47] Many cases of cryptogenic cirrhosis are actually end-stage NASH and currently account for 4% to 10% of liver transplants. Evidence shows that modest and sustained weight reduction, particularly in association with exercise, improves aminotransferase levels, reduces steatosis, and it also resolves steatohepatitis and reverses hepatic fibrosis.[48] "Crash dieting" or fasting must be avoided because precipitant and profound weight loss (greater than 2 lbs [1 kg]/week) is associated with worsening liver test abnormalities and accelerated hepatic fibrosis, or even liver failure.[49] Most patients who had a liver transplant between 1988 and 1996 were overweight (BMI >25 kg/m^2). Morbid obesity (BMI >40 kg/m^2) is associated with decreased 30-day, 1-year, and 2-year survival after liver transplant.[50] Many transplant programs will not offer liver transplantation to morbidly obese patients who have cirrhosis because of the reduced survival. Severe obesity is also associated with a reduced 5-year survival after liver transplantation. Hence, during regular office visits all obese patients must be strongly encouraged to have sustained weight loss.

Consumption of raw seafood should be avoided in patients with cirrhosis because of the risk of septicemia with *Vibrio vulnificus*. It is a species of halophilic gram-negative bacilli found in marine organisms and seawater. It can cause septicemia, which has a very high mortality rate of up to 50% when consumed with raw seafood. It can also cause a wound infection when the patient comes in contact with contaminated seawater.

ALCOHOL ABSTINENCE

More than 18 million adults in the United States abuse alcohol. Excessive alcohol intake is a common cause for liver cirrhosis in the western world, causing significant morbidity and mortality. Many of these patients have other psychiatric comorbidities along with alcohol problems.[51] Alcoholic patients have a higher incidence of anxiety disorders, affective disorders, and depression[52] as compared with nonalcoholic patients. These patients should be screened for these disorders at every visit.

Previous studies have shown that the risk for developing hepatocellular carcinoma (HCC) increases when daily consumption of alcohol exceeds 80 g/d for more than 10 years.[53] Most epidemiologic studies have shown that the effects of alcohol and the hepatitis C virus (HCV) on liver disease progression are synergistic. Case-control and cross-sectional studies have shown that the risk of developing HCC is higher in patients who continue to drink and have hepatitis C than patients with hepatitis C alone.[54] Patients who continue to drink and develop HCC have an increased risk for developing a poorly-differentiated HCC (confirmed at resection) as compared with patients who do not drink alcohol.[55] Tumor-free survival is also decreased in patients with HCV and alcohol. The same is true for alcohol consumption and hepatitis B infection. A longitudinal study from Japan had shown a 5-fold increase in the relative risk for HCC if a patient with hepatitis B continues to drink more than 27 g/d of alcohol.[56] Alcohol also increases the risk for both oral and pharyngeal cancer.

Consumption of alcohol decreases the response to interferon in patients with HCV.[57] Patients with cirrhosis have a much lesser response rate than patients without cirrhosis; hence every effort must be made to stop alcohol consumption before treatment with interferon. Preferably, these patients should be abstinent for at least 6 months before treatment.

Abstinence from alcohol can cause dramatic improvement in patients with even decompensated liver disease, and it can improve survival.[58] Most liver transplant programs require a 6 month period of abstinence and evaluation by a psychiatrist to address the issue of addiction before transplantation. Hence, every effort must be made to make sure that patients with advanced liver disease, especially those with decompensation, stop drinking alcohol. This requires counseling during office visits, outpatient alcohol rehabilitation, Alcoholics Anonymous support groups, and also the help of a psychologist and/or a psychiatrist.

TOBACCO ABSTINENCE

Tobacco use, particularly cigarette smoking, is the single most preventable cause of death in the United States. Cigarette smoking alone is directly responsible for approximately 30% of all cancer deaths annually in the United States.[59] Cigarette smoking also causes chronic lung disease (emphysema and chronic bronchitis), cardiovascular disease, stroke, and cataracts. Tobacco use is associated with an elevated risk for lung cancer and other cancers of the upper aerodigestive tract, stomach, liver, pancreas, bladder, kidney, and cervix, and also certain types of leukemia.

The liver is a natural target of many carcinogens in tobacco.[60] Several case-control studies have shown that there is a direct association of smoking and risk for liver cancer.[61] A synergistic effect for development of HCC in patients with chronic hepatitis B or C who continue to smoke is also present.[62] Patients with cirrhosis are at an increased risk for developing HCC, which may increase with the addition of tobacco. In patients with chronic hepatitis C, smoking was found to be independently associated with elevated liver enzyme levels and an increased fibrosis stage.[63]

Patients with cirrhosis can develop hypoxia because of the hepatopulmonary syndrome. It causes widespread intrapulmonary vasodilatation. Patients can have an abnormal gas exchange, which, if severe, may make them unsuitable candidates for liver transplantation. Smoking also causes several chronic lung diseases, like emphysema and chronic bronchitis. This, along with even mild to moderate hepatopulmonary syndrome, may make the patient severely hypoxic. Recent studies have shown that patients with moderate to severe hypoxia have an increased mortality rate after liver transplantation.[64]

Patients who have cirrhosis and smoke have an increased risk for developing hepatic artery thrombosis after transplantation if they continue to smoke.[65] This causes graft loss, biliary complications, sepsis, and even death. Tobacco consumption is a significant risk factor, together with pre–liver transplant alcohol intake, in the development of de novo tumors after liver transplantation.[66] Because of these reasons, many liver transplant programs will not offer liver transplantation to a patient who continues to smoke.

Smoking cessation has major and immediate health benefits for men and women of all ages. Quitting smoking decreases the risk for lung and other cancers, heart attack, stroke, and chronic lung disease. Hence, smoking cessation should strongly be advocated in all patients, especially for patients with cirrhosis. The benefits of smoking cessation should be discussed at every office visit. Nicotine replacement products deliver small, measured doses of nicotine into the body, which helps to relieve the cravings and withdrawal symptoms often felt by people trying to quit smoking. Strong and consistent evidence shows that nicotine replacement products can help people quit smoking.[67] There are several methods to help patients quit smoking. Nicotine is available in a patch, gum, lozenge, and even nasal spray. Bupropion, a prescription antidepressant marketed as Zyban, was approved by the FDA in 1997 to treat nicotine addiction. Varenicline, a prescription medicine marketed as Chantix, was also approved by the FDA in 2006 to help cigarette smokers stop smoking.

MANAGEMENT OF PAIN/USE OF ACETAMINOPHEN

Patients with liver disease may develop acute or chronic pain from a variety of causes. Advanced liver disease may lead to ascites causing abdominal and lower back pain. Chronic lower extremity edema causes pain, gynecomastia leads to mastalgia, and hepatocellular carcinoma when infiltrating the capsule becomes very painful. Management of pain in patients with liver cirrhosis and hepatic impairment remains a challenge. There are no available guidelines about the use of over-the-counter analgesics such as nonsteroidal antiinflammatory drugs (NSAIDs), acetaminophen, and most prescription drugs. Most medications and ingested substances pass through the liver for clearance, detoxification, and finally excretion. Altered liver function may enhance or predispose patients to drug toxicity.

In patients with cirrhosis and hepatic failure, the pharmacokinetics of opioids is affected in several different ways. The liver is the major site for biotransformation of most opioids, the major pathway being oxidation. When this is reduced, there is a decrease in drug clearance and increased oral bioavailability because of reduced first-pass metabolism.[68] There is a risk for the accumulation of the drug with repeat administrations. Patients with cirrhosis can have decreased creatinine clearance, causing the hydrophilic metabolites to accumulate. This may cause severe respiratory depression and may also precipitate hepatic encephalopathy. Metabolites of meperidine can accumulate, causing neurotoxic effects and seizures. Opioids should generally be avoided in these patients, but if needed should be used in the lowest dose possible with the longest possible interval between doses. Patients with cirrhosis need to be monitored very closely for any side effects of these medications, especially with respect to the impact on mentation. Tramadol is a centrally acting synthetic analgesic compound that is not derived from natural sources nor is it chemically related to opiates. Although its mode of action is not completely understood from animal tests, at least 2 complementary mechanisms appear applicable: binding to μ-opioid receptors and inhibition of reuptake of norepinephrine and serotonin. It has good analgesic properties and a short half-life of about 6 hrs. It appears to be safer than opioids; however, there have been no large studies proving its safety in cirrhosis.

Acetaminophen is a commonly used analgesic and has been in clinical use for more than 100 years. It lacks the inhibitory actions on platelet aggregation or the gastrointestinal toxicity of aspirin.[69] However, it can cause acute liver damage when massive doses are ingested. Patients with cirrhosis may have an altered metabolism, increased cytochrome P450 activity, and depleted glutathione stores.[70] This causes an increase in production of the hepatotoxic intermediate, N-acetyl-p-benzoquinone imine. Studies were done on the use of up to 4 g/d of acetaminophen for 13 days in patients (n = 20) with chronic liver disease.[71] There was no toxicity reported in any of the patients. In a more recent randomized, double-blind, placebo-controlled study, the safety of acetaminophen in patients with hepatitis C was shown.[72] There was no effect on serum levels of alanine aminotransferase when up to 3 g/d of acetaminophen was used for 7 days in these patients. Chronic alcohol consumption has been associated with decreased glutathione levels and is thought to increase the risk of acetaminophen hepatotoxicity.[73,74] It appears that the use of acetaminophen in doses of up to 2 g/d is safe in patients with cirrhosis who are not actively drinking alcohol.[75] Acetaminophen, or any products containing it, should not be used in any patient with cirrhosis who continues to consume alcohol.

NSAIDs can be more toxic to patients with cirrhosis because of 2 mechanisms. Patients with cirrhosis have impaired coagulation and bleeding tendencies. NSAIDs cause impairment in platelet function and aggregation which can cause further bleeding. Renal prostaglandin production is blocked, which may cause a decrease in renal blood flow and lead to renal failure. Hence, NSAIDs should be avoided in patients with cirrhosis. In reduced dosages, acetaminophen appears to be a safe alternative in patients with cirrhosis who do not drink alcohol.

USE OF MEDICATIONS

Drug-induced hepatotoxicity increases in patients with cirrhosis. Most prescription and nonprescription medications pass through the liver for clearance, detoxification, and eventual excretion. These mechanisms can be impaired in patients with cirrhosis. The reported incidence of drug-induced hepatotoxicity is between 1 in 10,000 and 1 in 100,000 healthy patients.[76] This is increased in patients with cirrhosis; however, the true incidence is difficult to determine because of underreporting and missed diagnosis. The factors that increase the risk for drug-induced liver injury include dose, duration of treatment, older age, female gender, genetic predisposition,[77] and underlying liver disease.

Several mechanisms involved in causing drug-related toxicity in patients with cirrhosis have been discussed. Impaired production of albumin results in reduced plasma binding of several drugs and thus increases availability of the circulating drug pool for tissue uptake and pharmacodynamic effects.[78] Impaired secretion of bile acids, bilirubin, and other organic anions is seen in cirrhosis, which could be responsible for impaired biliary excretion of drugs and their metabolites.[79] Portal-systemic shunting, which is common in advanced liver cirrhosis, substantially decreases the presystemic elimination (ie, first-pass effect) of high extraction drugs following their oral administration, thus leading to a significant increase in the extent of absorption. The activity of the various CYP450 enzymes seems differentially affected in patients with cirrhosis. Glucuronidation is often affected to a lesser extent than CYP450-mediated reactions in mild to moderate cirrhosis but can be substantially impaired in patients with advanced cirrhosis.[80]

Dosage adjustment in patients with liver dysfunction is essential for many drugs to avoid excessive accumulation of the drug, and possibly of active drug metabolite(s), which may lead to serious adverse reactions. Drugs must be given with caution to patients with severe hepatic insufficiency, which can be the case in cirrhosis. Before administering drugs that are largely eliminated by hepatic mechanisms, the potential therapeutic benefits must be carefully counterbalanced with the risk for serious toxic reactions. The patient's hepatologist should be made aware of any new medications which have a potential to cause further liver damage and hepatotoxicity. Patients with cirrhosis should discuss the safety of all prescribed and over-the-counter medications with the hepatologist before starting a new medication.

Box 1
Recommendations for cirrhotic patients

1. Discuss and clear all medications (both prescribed and over-the-counter) with my office before taking them.

2. Do not take aspirin/NSAIDs/COX-2 inhibitors without a discussion with my office.

3. Acetaminophen can be used at a dose of 2 g daily (such as 500 mg every 6 hours, or 1,000 mg every 12 hours) so long as you are not drinking alcohol.

4. Do not eat raw seafood or shellfish.

5. Only swim in chlorinated water—avoid swimming in ocean water.

6. Discuss and clear all elective surgery with my office, given the risk for surgery in patients with cirrhosis.

7. Be sure to be vaccinated against the flu (influenza) each year, have the pneumococcal vaccine once, and the Td vaccine every 10 years.

8. Make sure you are screened every 6 months for the development of liver cancer (hepatocellular carcinoma) with both a blood test (such as alpha-fetoprotein or AFP) and an imaging study (ultrasound, MRI, or CT scan).

9. Call my office and go to the ER for evaluation if any of the following occur:

   a) Temperature greater than 101°F.

   b) Confusion.

   c) Vomiting blood.

   d) Rectal bleeding.

   e) Vomiting more than once during a 24-hour period.

   f) Abdominal or chest pain.

   g) Shortness of breath.

   h) Blood in the urine.

   i) Development or worsening of jaundice.

   j) Development or worsening of lower extremity edema or ascites (fluid in the abdomen).

   k) Diarrhea.

10. Please inform our office if you are being seen in the ER or admitted to the hospital.

11. Please have the ER physician contact our office to assist in your evaluation during your visit to the ER.

12. Know the dosages of all of your medications, and how often you take them, especially if you are on diuretics or being treated for hepatic encephalopathy.

WHEN TO SEEK MEDICAL ATTENTION

Patients with cirrhosis should contact their physicians when they are ill. In addition to being immunocompromised, they are unable to tolerate dehydration. It is our practice to discuss with each patient who has cirrhosis the clinical implications of having cirrhosis, either at their initial visit or once they have progressed to cirrhosis. It is explained, in simple terms, that they should not stay home when they are sick. All

---

Box 2
When to go to the emergency room

Having cirrhosis puts patients at increased risk when they get sick. Do not stay home when you are ill. Patients with cirrhosis are at an increased risk for infections and have difficulties fighting infections. If warranted, it is very important to be treated with antibiotics as soon as possible. Patients with cirrhosis have a hard time tolerating dehydration, so it is important that intravenous fluids be given as soon as possible if a patient is at risk for dehydration.

You should call the office and go to the ER for evaluation if any of the following occur:

a) Temperature greater than 101°F.

b) Confusion.

c) Vomiting blood.

d) Rectal bleeding.

e) Vomiting more than once during a 24-hour period.

f) Abdominal or chest pain.

g) Shortness of breath.

h) Blood in the urine.

i) Development or worsening of jaundice.

j) Development or worsening of lower extremity edema or ascites (fluid in the abdomen).

k) Diarrhea.

You should call 911 if confusion or gastrointestinal bleeding occurs!

WHEN YOU ARRIVE AT THE EMERGENCY ROOM
Once you arrive at the ER, please have the ER physician call our office and ask to speak with your hepatologist. There are always a Gastroenterology (GI) Fellow and a hepatologist on-call 24 hours a day/7 days a week. The telephone number is 215-xxx-xxxx. Ask for the GI Fellow on call.
Give this paper to the nurse and physician taking care of you in the ER.

Dear Emergency Room Physician,

This patient has cirrhosis. If this patient has arrived at your ER because of either a fever or confusion, we would recommend that you obtain the following tests:

1. CBC with differential, SMA7, LFTs, PT/INR.

2. CXR (PA and lateral).

3. Urinalysis and culture

4. Blood cultures

5. Sputum cultures (if applicable)

Please call our office at the above number so that we can discuss this patient's case in detail.
Sincerely,

Kenneth D. Rothstein, MD.

patients with cirrhosis are given a list of signs and symptoms (**Box 1**) for which they should seek medical attention. This involves a visit to the local ER and a call to our office. Prompt identification and treatment of infection can be lifesaving. Infections can present without fever, but only with a change in mental status. Vomiting and diarrhea need to be treated along with fluid resuscitation before dehydration leads to hypotension. Patients with cirrhosis are advised to contact our office if they are being seen in the ER or have been admitted to the hospital. Communication between ER physicians and the hepatologist is crucial, since the management of patients with cirrhosis in the ER requires special care. Our patients with cirrhosis are given a handout that should be given to the ER to help facilitate their care (**Box 2**). Strict adherence to the recommendations should help to minimize the morbidity and mortality of cirrhosis.

SUMMARY

Maintaining a healthy lifestyle and good preventative strategies in patients with cirrhosis is extremely important. This may not only prevent decompensation in patients with cirrhosis but also may slow down the progression of the underlying liver disease. These individuals already have compromised liver function and any additional insult may be detrimental to their health. Preventive maneuvers may not only prevent the need for liver transplantation but also prevent death. Appropriate vaccination, screening for osteoporosis, and abstinence from alcohol and tobacco are all critically important interventions in these patients. Special care should be given to maintain adequate nutrition. Adequate pain control with appropriate medication is essential for maintaining quality of life in this patient population. All this can be achieved with coordination between the patient's hepatologist and primary care physician.

REFERENCES

1. National Center for Health Statistics. National vital statistics report. Chronic liver disease/cirrhosis. Available at: www.cdc.gov/nchs/fastats/liverdis.htm. Accessed November 2008.
2. Riley TR III, Bhatti AM. Preventive strategies in chronic liver disease: part II. Cirrhosis. Am Fam Physician 2001;64:1735–40.
3. Sandler RS, Everhart JE, Doniwitz M, et al. The burden of selective digestive disease in the United States. Gastroenterology 2002;122:1500–11.
4. Disease burden from viral hepatitis A, B and C in the United States. Atlanta (GA): Centers for Disease Control and Prevention; 2002.
5. Williams I, Bell B, Kaluba J, et al. Association between chronic liver disease and death from hepatitis A, United States, 1989–92 [Abstract no. A39]. IX Triennial International Symposium on Viral Hepatitis and Liver Disease. Rome, Italy, April 21–25, 1996.
6. Stapleton JT. Host immune response to hepatitis A virus. J Infect Dis 1995; 171(Suppl 1):S9–14.
7. Akriviadis EA, Redeker AG. Fulminant hepatitis A in intravenous drug users with chronic liver disease. Ann Intern Med 1989;110:838–9.
8. Lee SD, Chan CY, Yu MI, et al. Safety and immunogenicity of inactivated hepatitis A vaccine in patients with chronic liver disease. J Med Virol 1997;52:215–8.
9. Available at: http://www.cdc.gov/hepatitis/statistics.htm. Accessed November 2008.
10. Mast EE, Margolis HS, Fiore AE, et al. A comprehensive immunization strategy to eliminate transmission of hepatitis B virus infection in the United States. MMWR Recomm Rep 2005;54:1–31.

11. Poland GA. Hepatitis B immunization in health care workers: dealing with vaccine nonresponse. Am J Prev Med 1998;15:73–7.

12. Hepatitis B virus: a comprehensive strategy for eliminating transmission in the United States through universal childhood vaccination. MMWR Recomm Rep 1991;40:1–25.

13. Katz SL, LaMontagne J, Hardegree C. FDA approval for a combined hepatitis A and B vaccine. MMWR Morb Mortal Wkly Rep 2001;50:806–7.

14. Thompson WW, Shay DK, Weintraub E, et al. Influenza-associated hospitalizations in the United States. JAMA 2004;292:1333–40.

15. Gross PA, Russo C, Dran S, et al. Time to earliest peak serum antibody response to influenza vaccine in the elderly. Clin Diagn Lab Immunol 1997;4:491–2.

16. CDC. Pneumococcal polysaccharide vaccine usage, United States. MMWR Morb Mortal Wkly Rep 1984;33:273–6, 281.

17. Hay JE. Osteoporosis in liver diseases and after liver transplantation. J Hepatol 2003;38:856–65.

18. Carey EJ, Balan V, Kremers WK, et al. Osteopenia and osteoporosis in patients with end-stage liver disease caused by hepatitis C and alcoholic liver disease: not just a cholestatic problem. Liver Transpl 2003;9:1166–73.

19. Guichelarr M, Hay J, Clark B, et al. Pretransplant bone histomorphometric status of patients with end-stage liver cholestatic liver disease. J Hepatol 2000;32:54.

20. Crosbie O, Freaney R, McKenna MJ, et al. Bone density, vitamin D status and disordered bone remodeling in end-stage chronic liver disease. Calcif Tissue Int 1999;64:295–300.

21. Diamond T, Stiel D, Lunzer M, et al. Osteoporosis and skeletal fractures in chronic liver disease. Gut 1990;31:82–7.

22. Sokhi RP, Anantharaju A, Kondaveeti R, et al. Bone mineral density among cirrhotic patients awaiting liver transplantation. Liver Transpl 2004;10:648–53.

23. Janes CH, Dickson ER, Okazaki R, et al. Role of hyperbilirubinemia in the impairment of osteoblast proliferation associated with cholestatic jaundice. J Clin Invest 1995;95:2581–6.

24. Cemborain A, Castilla-Cortazar I, Garcia M, et al. Osteopenia in rats with liver cirrhosis: beneficial effects of IGF-1 treatment. J Hepatol 1998;28:122–31.

25. Angulo P, Batts KP, Jorgensen RA, et al. Oral budesonide in the treatment of primary sclerosing cholangitis. Am J Gastroenterol 2000;31:318–23.

26. Kurihara N, Roodman GD. Interferons-alpha and gamma inhibit interleukin-1 beta stimulated osteoclast-like cell formation in the long term human marrow cultures. J Interferon Res 1990;10:541–7.

27. Compston JE. Hepatic osteodystrophy: vitamin D metabolism in patients with liver disease. Gut 1986;27:1073–90.

28. Epstein S. The roles of bone mineral density, bone turnover, and other properties in reducing fracture risk during antiresorptive therapy. Mayo Clin Proc 2005;80: 379–88.

29. Floreani A, Zappala F, Naccarato R, et al. A 3 year pilot study with 1,25-dihydroxyvitamin D, calcium, and calcitonin for severe osteodystrophy in PBC. J Clin Gastroenterol 1997;24:239–44.

30. Fitzpatrick L. Selective estrogen receptor modulators and phytoestrogens: new therapies for the postmenopausal women. Mayo Clin Proc 1999;74:601–7.

31. NIH consensus development panel on optimal calcium intake. Optimal calcium intake. JAMA 1994;272:1942–8.

32. Mobarhan S, Russell R, Recker RR, et al. Metabolic bone disease in alcoholic cirrhosis. Hepatology 1984;4:266–73.

33. Romijn JA, Klein S. Extra hepatic metabolic consequences of cirrhosis. Gastroenterology 1999;102:2175–7.
34. Italian Multicentric Cooperative Project in nutrition in liver cirrhosis. Nutritional status in cirrhosis. J Hepatol 1994;21:317–25.
35. Scolapio JS, Ukleja A, McGreevy K, et al. Nutritional problems in end-stage liver disease: contribution of impaired gastric emptying and ascites. J Clin Gastroenterol 2002;34(1):89–93.
36. Madden AM, Bradbury W, Morgan MY. Taste perception in cirrhosis; its relationship to circulating micronutrients and food preferences. Hepatology 1997;26:40–8.
37. Testa R, Franceschini R, Giannini E. Serum leptin levels in patients with viral chronic hepatitis or liver cirrhosis. J Hepatol 2000;33:33–7.
38. Vlahcevic ZR, Buhac I, Farrar JJ, et al. Bile acid metabolism in patients with cirrhosis. Gastroenterology 1971;60:491–8.
39. Galati JS, Holderman KP, Bottjen PL, et al. Gastric emptying and orocecal transit in portal hypertension and end-stage chronic liver disease. Liver Transpl Surg 1997;3:34–8.
40. Romijn JA, Endert E, Sauerwein HP. Glucose and fat metabolism during short-term starvation in cirrhosis. Gastroenterology 1991;100:731–7.
41. Zoli M, Marchesini G, Dondi C, et al. Myofibrillar protein catabolic rates in cirrhotic patients with and without muscle wasting. Clin Sci 1982;62:683–6.
42. Fiqueiredo F, Dickson ER, Pasha T, et al. Impact of nutritional status on outcomes after liver transplantation. Transplantation 2000;70(9):1347–52.
43. Orloff MJ, Charters AC, Chandler JG, et al. Portacaval shunt as emergency procedure in patients with alcoholic cirrhosis. Surg Gynecol Obstet 1975;141:59–68.
44. Leevy CM, Davison E. Portal hypertension and hepatic coma. Postgrad Med J 1967;41:84–93.
45. Weber FL, Minco D, Fresard KM, et al. Effects of vegetable diets on nitrogen metabolism in cirrhotic subjects. Gastroenterology 1985;89:538–44.
46. Ritter DM, Rettke SR, Hughes RW, et al. Placement of nasogastric tubes and esophageal stethoscopes in patients with documented esophageal varices. Anesth Analg 1988;67:283–5.
47. Adler M, Schaffner F. Fatty liver hepatitis and cirrhosis in obese patients. Am J Med 1979;67:811–6.
48. Hickman IJ, Jonsson JR, Prins JB, et al. Modest weight loss and physical activity in overweight patients with chronic liver disease results in sustained improvements in alanine aminotransferase, fasting insulin, and quality of life. Gut 2004;53:413–9.
49. Caldwell SH, Hespenheide EE. Subacute liver failure in obese women. Am J Gastroenterol 2002;97:2058–62.
50. Nair S, Verma S, Thuluvant PJ. Obesity and its effects on survival in patients undergoing orthotopic liver transplantation in United States. Hepatology 2002;35:105–9.
51. Marshall EJ, Alam F. Psychiatric problems associated with alcohol misuse and dependence. Br J Hosp Med 1997;58:44–6.
52. Schuckit MA, Hesselbrock V. Alcohol dependence and anxiety disorders: what is the relationship? Am J Psychiatry 1994;151:1723–34.
53. Donato F, Tagger A, Gelatti U. Alcohol and hepatocellular carcinoma: the effect of lifetime intake and hepatitis virus infections in men and women. Am J Epidemiol 2002;36:1206–13.
54. De Bac C, Stroffolini T, Gaeta GB. Pathogenic factors in cirrhosis with and without hepatocellular carcinoma: a multicenter Italian study. Hepatology 1994;20:1225–30.

55. Kubo S, Kinoshita H, Hirohashi K. High malignancy of hepatocellular carcinoma in alcoholic patients with hepatitis C virus. Surgery 1997;121:425–9.

56. Oshima A, Tsukuma H, Hiyama T, et al. Follow-up study of HBsAg-positive blood donors with special reference to effect of drinking and smoking on development of liver cancer. Int J Cancer 1984;34:775–9.

57. Peters MG, Terrault NA. Alcohol use and hepatitis C. Hepatology 2002;36(Suppl 1): S220–5.

58. Powell WJ, Klatskin G. Duration and survival in patients with Laennec's cirrhosis. Am J Med 1968;44:406–20.

59. Centers for Disease Control and Prevention. Annual smoking-attributable mortality, years of potential life lost, and productivity losses—United States, 1997–2001. MMWR Morb Mortal Wkly Rep 2005;54:625–8.

60. Mant JWF, Vessey MP. Trends in mortality from primary liver cancer in England and Wales 1975–92: influence of oral contraceptives. Br J Cancer 1995;72: 800–3.

61. Marrero JA, Fontana RJ, Fu S, et al. Alcohol, tobacco and obesity are synergistic risk factors for hepatocellular carcinoma. J Hepatol 2005;42:218–24.

62. Kuper H, Tzonou A, Kaklamani E, et al. Tobacco smoking, alcohol consumption and their interaction in the causation of hepatocellular carcinoma. Int J Cancer 2000;85(4):498–502.

63. Hezode C, Lonjon I, Roudot-Thoraval F, et al. Impact of smoking on histological lever lesions in chronic hepatitis C. Gut 2003;52:126–9.

64. Arguedas MR, Abrams GA, Krowka MJ, et al. Prospective evaluation of outcomes and predictors of mortality in patients with hepatopulmonary syndrome under-going liver transplantation. Hepatology 2003;37:192–7.

65. Pungpapong S, Reich DJ, Rothstein KD, et al. Cigarette smoking is associated with an increase incidence of vascular complications after liver transplantation. Liver Transpl 2002;8:582–7.

66. Catalina MV, de Diego A, García-Sánchez A, et al. Characterization of de novo malignancies in liver transplantation. Gastroenterol Hepatol 2003;26:57–63.

67. Fiore MC, Bailey WC, Cohen SJ, et al. Smoking cessation: agency for health care policy and research, US department of health and human services. Agency for Health Care Policy and Research; 1996.

68. Tegeder I, Geisslinger G, Lotsch J, et al. Therapy with opioids in liver or renal failure. Schmerz 1999;13(3):183–95.

69. Koch-Weser J. Drug therapy. Acetaminophen. N Engl J Med 1976;295:1297–300.

70. Benson GD. Hepatotoxicity following the therapeutic use of antipyretic analgesics. Am J Med 1983;75:85–93.

71. Benson GD. Acetaminophen in chronic liver disease. Clin Pharmacol Ther 1983; 33:95–101.

72. Dargere S, Collet T, Crampon D, et al. Lack of toxicity of acetaminophen in patients with chronic hepatitis C. Gastroenterology 2000;118:A947.

73. Burgunder J-M, Lauterburg BH. Decreased production of glutathione in patients with cirrhosis. Eur J Clin Invest 1987;17:408–14.

74. Jewell SA, Di Monte D, Gentile A, et al. Decreased hepatic glutathione in chronic alcoholic patients. J Hepatol 1986;3:1–6.

75. Riley TR, Smith JP. Preventive care in chronic liver disease. J Gen Intern Med 1999;14:699–704.

76. Larrey D. Epidemiology and individual susceptibility to adverse drug reactions affecting the liver. Semin Liver Dis 2002;22:145–55.

77. Larrey D, Pageaux GP. Genetic predisposition to drug-induced hepatotoxicity. J Hepatol 1997;26(Suppl 2):12–21.

78. MacKichan JJ. Influence of protein binding and use of unbound (free) drug concentrations. In: Burton ME, Shaw LM, Schentag JJ, et al, editors. Applied pharmacokinetics & pharmacodynamics—principles of therapeutic drug monitoring. Philadelphia: Lippincott Williams & Wilkins; 2006. p. 82–120.

79. Traumer M, Meier PJ, Boyer JL. Molecular regulation of hepatocellular transport systems in cholestasis. J Hepatol 1999;31:165–78.

80. Chalasani N, Gorski JC, Patel NH, et al. Hepatic and intestinal cytochrome P450 3A activity in cirrhosis: effects of transjugular intrahepatic portosystemic shunts. Hepatology 2001;34:1103–8.

Preoperative Risk Assessment for Patients with Liver Disease

Shahid M. Malik, MD, Jawad Ahmad, MD, MRCP*

KEYWORDS

- Operative risk • Liver disease • Cirrhosis
- CTP score • MELD

Underlying liver disease has effects on the risk of morbidity and mortality after surgery. The magnitude of the risk depends on several factors, including the etiology and severity of liver disease, the surgical procedure, and the type of anesthesia used.

In patients with cirrhosis, nontransplant surgery can lead to worsening of underlying liver disease or even liver failure. The reasons for this are unclear but may reflect circulatory changes brought on by surgery or anesthesia, resulting in impaired hepatic vascular flow.

The number of patients with advanced liver disease is on the increase, and so the number of patients with liver disease who will require surgery will likely increase. It is not uncommon for patients with liver disease to undergo surgical interventions other than liver transplant. Up to 10% of patients with advanced liver disease require a surgical procedure in the final 2 years of their life.[1]

Identification of the surgical risk is important in every patient; however, the risk assessment in patients with liver disease is imperative and can be lifesaving. Gastroenterologists and hepatologists are frequently asked to evaluate patients with liver disease and determine their risk of undergoing surgical procedures and to help make recommendations that may optimize outcomes.

PREOPERATIVE SCREENING FOR LIVER DISEASE

The primary goal of preoperative screening is to determine the presence of preexisting liver disease using the least invasive means possible.

The value of a thorough history and physical examination cannot be overestimated. It is crucial in providing clues as to whether a patient has liver disease or is at an increased risk of having liver disease. All patients should be questioned regarding prior

Division of Gastroenterology, Hepatology and Nutrition, University of Pittsburgh School of Medicine, Pittsburgh, PA 15213, USA
* Corresponding author.
E-mail address: ahmadj@msx.upmc.edu (J. Ahmad).

Med Clin N Am 93 (2009) 917–929
doi:10.1016/j.mcna.2009.03.001
0025-7125/09/$ – see front matter © 2009 Elsevier Inc. All rights reserved.

remote blood transfusions, tattoos, illicit drug use, alcohol intake, sexual history, personal history of jaundice, and family history of liver disease. A complete review of medications, including over-the-counter analgesics and complementary or alternative medications should also be sought. Complaints of excessive fatigue, pruritus, and easy bruisability may be indicators of underlying liver dysfunction. Physical examination can identify signs that are consistent with chronic underlying liver disease, such as the presence of jaundice, palmar erythema, spider telangiectasia, parotid gland enlargement, Dupuytren contracture, hepatosplenomegaly, ascites, dilated abdominal veins, lower extremity edema, gynecomastia, testicular atrophy, temporal wasting, or loss of muscle mass.

Patients who are deemed healthy without clinical suspicion for underlying liver disease generally do not require laboratory testing of liver function. A study from 1976, in which 7620 subjects undergoing elective surgery were screened with blood work, revealed that only 11 had abnormal liver tests.[2] Although this study preceded the current epidemics in viral hepatitis and fatty liver disease, it supports the notion that routine screening without clinical suspicion of underlying liver disease is of low yield and would likely not improve outcomes.

If the liver function tests are found to be abnormal, then it is prudent to defer elective surgery until a more thorough investigation can be performed to determine the nature, chronicity, and severity of the biochemical abnormalities. For those patients who are asymptomatic with only mild elevations in aminotransferases and normal total bilirubin concentration, cancellation of surgery is rarely required. If, however, patients are found to have elevated aminotransferase levels greater than 3 times the upper limits of normal or abnormalities in parameters of synthetic function (namely bilirubin and prothrombin time), further investigation is warranted. The incidence of underlying cirrhosis in patients with abnormal liver function tests has been reported to be anywhere from 6% to 34%.[3,4] Further investigation in this subgroup of patients should proceed along standard pathways for the workup of chronic liver disease. Investigations should include viral hepatitis serology for hepatitis B and C, specific tests for metabolic liver disease, such as iron studies for hemochromatosis, ceruloplasmin level for Wilson disease, α1-antitrypsin level and phenotyping, serum markers for autoimmune liver disease, and imaging, such as a right upper quadrant ultrasound with Doppler to evaluate the hepatic parenchyma, biliary system, and flow within the portal venous vasculature, and CT or MRI scan for evidence of cirrhosis or portal hypertension (**Fig. 1**).

Once it has been determined that a patient has liver disease, the next step is estimating the risk of surgery. Patients with liver disease are at a greater risk for surgical and anesthetic complications than those without liver disease.[5–7] The degree of risk associated with the surgery and postoperative outcomes is largely dependent on 3 factors: the etiology and severity of the liver disease, the specific surgery planned, and the type of anesthesia (**Fig. 2**).

NATURE OF THE UNDERLYING LIVER DISEASE

Because of the high perioperative morbidity and mortality, acute hepatitis is regarded as a contraindication to elective surgery (**Box 1**). This recommendation is largely based upon older literature, in which patients with icteric hepatitis had a 10% to 13% mortality following laparotomy.[8,9] The increased risk is likely the result of acute hepatocellular injury, inflammation, and associated hepatic dysfunction. If the degree of liver injury is severe, consideration should be given to delay even urgent surgery. Most cases of acute hepatitis are self-limited and so surgery should be postponed

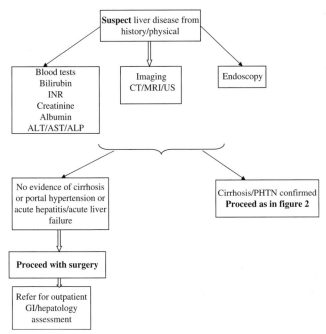

Fig. 1. Algorithm for preoperative assessment in patients with suspected liver disease.

until the patient's clinical, biochemical, and histological parameters return to normal. Improvement in the underlying condition, whether it is viral, toxic, drug induced, thrombotic, or hypoxic, will likely reduce postoperative risk.

The specific case of acute alcoholic hepatitis deserves special mention. The presentation of acute alcoholic hepatitis (jaundice, right upper quadrant pain, elevated liver function tests, and leukocytosis) can many times mimic an acute biliary process, and lead to misdiagnosis and subsequent "therapeutic misadventures," namely, cholecystectomy or endoscopic retrograde cholangiopancreatography , with devastating postoperative results.[10] All elective surgeries should be delayed in patients with acute alcoholic hepatitis until clinical and laboratory parameters return to normal.

Patients with mild chronic hepatitis without evidence of portal hypertension and well-preserved hepatic function generally tolerate surgery well.[11] However, when the disease is considered active, evidenced by clinical, biochemical, and histological measures, surgical risk increases.[6] When a patient with chronic hepatitis has evidence of clinical decompensation (impaired hepatic synthesis, altered excretion, portal hypertension), the perioperative risk is higher.[11–13] It is unclear whether interventions aimed at improving active disease in these patients will help to improve outcomes after surgery.

Patients with well-compensated cirrhosis, but significant portal hypertension, may still be at increased risk of postoperative decompensation, particularly if the surgery involves the liver, such as resection of a tumor.[14] Limited data suggest that correction of the portal pressure by transjugular intrahepatic portosystemic shunt (TIPS) may reduce this risk in patients undergoing abdominal surgery.[15]

With the epidemic rise in the metabolic syndrome, more patients are presenting for surgery with nonalcoholic fatty liver disease (NAFLD). In one study, which included patients with alcoholic and nonalcoholic steatohepatitis with moderate steatosis

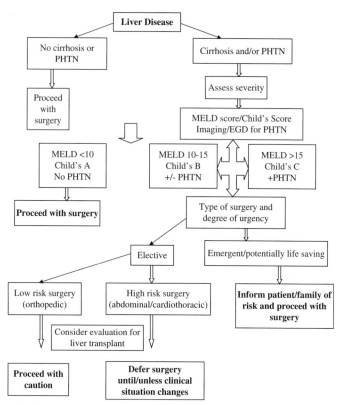

Fig. 2. Algorithm for preoperative assessment in patients with known liver disease.

(defined by >30% fat on liver biopsy) undergoing major hepatic resection, there was a trend towards increased morbidity and mortality following major hepatic resection.[16] These patients tended to be obese (mean body mass index >30 kg/m^2) with elevated total bilirubin levels (mean 2.2 mg/dL), indicating a degree of hepatic dysfunction. How much the steatosis alone contributed to the increased risk is unclear.

NAFLD is a common finding in patients undergoing bariatric surgery and typically improves after significant weight loss. Occasionally cirrhosis is found at the time of surgery, and increased perioperative mortality has been observed in this situation,[17] leading some surgeons to abort gastric bypass if frank cirrhosis is noted.

Box 1
High-risk patients with liver disease for any type of surgery

Child's C

MELD score greater than 15

Acute liver failure

Acute alcoholic hepatitis

High serum bilirubin (>11 mg/dL)

Obstructive jaundice has been shown to markedly increase perioperative mortality. Studies have suggested that patients with obstructive jaundice and risk factors including total bilirubin level greater than 11mg/dL, presence of malignancy, serum creatinine 1.4 mg/dL or more, blood urea nitrogen concentration greater than 10 mg/dL, albumin concentration less than 3 g/dL, initial hematocrit less than 30%, aspartate aminotransferase greater than 90 IU/L, and age more than 65 years, portend worse outcome following surgery.[18–20] Efforts to improve the jaundice either with endoscopic or percutaneous biliary drainage do not appear to improve mortality.[21–25] This suggests that severe underlying disease (cirrhosis or malignancy) is present in most patients, and relieving the jaundice does not change the natural history of the disease process.

CIRRHOSIS AND PREDICTIVE MODELS

Of patients with liver disease, the outcomes of those with cirrhosis have been studied most extensively. Once a patient has developed cirrhosis, grading the severity of the liver disease is of crucial importance in determining their perioperative risk.

Two scoring systems, the Model for End-Stage Liver Disease (MELD) (**Box 2**) and the Child-Turcotte-Pugh (CTP) classification (**Table 1**) have been adapted and evaluated to help clinicians determine perioperative morbidity and mortality in patients with cirrhosis undergoing surgical procedures.

The CTP was originally formulated by Child and Turcotte in 1964 to help predict mortality following portocaval shunt surgery.[26] This was modified a decade later by Pugh and colleagues,[27] who replaced nutritional status with prothrombin time and devised a scoring system for patients undergoing esophageal transections for bleeding varices.

The CTP score was the first-used predictor of surgical risk in patients with liver disease. Although the scoring system has never been prospectively validated, it is regarded to be an accurate predictor and is still widely used today to predict perioperative morbidity and mortality for elective and emergency surgeries in patients with cirrhosis.

The commonly quoted percentages linking perioperative mortality and CTP class are based largely upon two retrospective studies of patients with cirrhosis. Garrison and colleagues[1] studied 100 patients with cirrhosis who underwent abdominal surgery. Thirty patients died and major complications occurred in another 30 patients. Fifty-two variables were analyzed and in multivariate analysis, the CTP classification was the best predictor of morbidity and mortality with CTP class A, B, and C

Box 2
MELD score equation

MELD score = $(9.6 \times \log_e[\text{creatinine}]) + (3.8 \times \log_e[\text{bilirubin}]) + (11.2 \times \log_e[\text{INR}]) + 6.4$

Value of creatinine, bilirubin, or INR cannot be less than 1.0 for the equation.

Values greater than 40 assigned a value of 40.

MELD less than 10—consider low risk

MELD 10 to 15—intermediate risk

MELD greater than 15—high risk

Creatinine in mg/dL

Bilirubin in mg/dL

Table 1
Child-Turcotte-Pugh classification of cirrhosis

Clinical Trait	1 Point	2 Points	3 Points
Ascites	None	Present	Moderate/severe
Encephalopathy	None	Grade 1–2	Grade 3–4
Bilirubin (mg/dL)	<2	2–3	>3
Albumin (g/dL)	>3.5	2.8–3.5	<2.8
INR	<1.7	1.7–2.3	>2.3

The CTP score uses 5 variables and assigns point values according to severity. The composite score is between 5 (well compensated disease) and 15 (severe decompensation).
Child's A 5–6 points.
Child's B 7–9 points.
Child's C 10–15 points.

corresponding to postoperative mortality of 10%, 31%, and 76% (**Table 2**). In another study involving 92 cirrhotic patients, Mansour and colleagues[28] commented that the most accurate predictor of outcomes in patients with cirrhosis was Child's class with mortality percentages nearly identical to those quoted by Garrison and colleagues[1] with CTP A, B, and C corresponding to 10%, 30%, and 82%. In a larger review, spanning nearly 10 years, it was determined that cirrhotic patients undergoing any surgical procedure under anesthesia had perioperative mortality rates of 11.6% and complication rates of 30.1%. Mortality and complication rates correlated directly with the Child score.[29]

One of the drawbacks of the CTP classification is its partly subjective nature. Parameters such as grades of encephalopathy and degree of ascites are left to the discrepancy of the clinician. The need for a more accurate model to assess patients with liver disease was highlighted by Malinchoc and colleagues to predict outcome following TIPS. In this landmark study, the investigators formulated the MELD scoring system to help predict short-term mortality in patients with cirrhosis undergoing TIPS.[30] The MELD score incorporates three biochemical measurements into a complex logarithmic formula—the total bilirubin concentration, serum creatinine, and the international normalized ratio (INR). Patient scores range from 6 to 40, with 6 reflecting "early" disease and 40 "severe" disease. In 2002, the MELD score was adopted by the United Network for Organ Sharing as a means of more fairly allocating donor organs to ensure priority to the "sickest" recipients.

Table 2
CTP score and MELD score and risk of mortality after surgery

Type of Surgery	CTP/MELD Score	Mortality (%)
Abdominal	A	10
	B	30–31
	C	76–82
Cardiac	A	0–11
	B	18–50
	C	67–100
Abdominal/cardiac/orthopedic (30-d mortality)	<8	5.7
	>20	>50

The MELD score has been validated in a number of prospective studies as a prognostic score in determining mortality in patients with cirrhosis, acute variceal bleeding, acute alcoholic hepatitis, and acute liver failure.[31–36] The MELD score has also been examined as a prognostic tool in determining mortality following surgery.

One of the first studies to evaluate MELD score and postoperative outcomes involved 33 patients with cirrhosis undergoing laparoscopic cholecystectomy.[37] Two patients died in the study group versus none in noncirrhotic controls. The authors concluded that a MELD score of 8 or more identified patients at risk for postoperative morbidity following cholecystectomy. Several studies have since evaluated the usefulness of the MELD score in predicting perioperative morbidity and mortality.[38–41] These studies involved elective and emergent surgeries including abdominal, cardiac, and hepatic resection and orthopedic procedures. The type of surgery performed plays a large role in determining outcome, and so it is difficult to apply such studies to individual patients. A recent large study of almost 800 cirrhotic patients undergoing major digestive, orthopedic, or cardiac surgery demonstrated that the MELD score correlated with short-term and long-term mortality extending out to 20 years. For each point increase in the MELD score above 8, there was a 14% increase in 30- and 90-day mortality.[42] Overall, the MELD score correlates well with postoperative mortality and in some cases is superior to CTP class.

It has been recommended that patients with MELD scores below 10 can undergo elective surgery, whereas caution needs to be taken for patients with MELD scores between 10 and 15. For patients with MELD scores above 15, elective surgery should be avoided. It is most prudent in this group of patients to consider evaluation for liver transplant listing, in case the patient should decompensate post procedure.[43]

TYPE OF SURGERY

Studies have shown that patients with cirrhosis who undergo any type of emergency surgery (especially abdominal) have a higher mortality than patients with normal liver function (**Box 3**).

Emergency surgeries obviously do not permit for delays in the decision to intervene. Emergent surgeries, as the name implies, are life-threatening and many times must be undertaken irrespective of the patient's comorbidities. Patients with cirrhosis who require emergent surgical procedures have extremely high mortality rates. One study in which 14 patients with cirrhosis underwent emergent surgical procedures under general anesthesia showed a 1- and 3-month mortality of 19% and 44%, respectively,

---

Box 3
High-risk surgery in patients with liver disease

Abdominal surgery

Cholecystectomy

Colectomy

Gastric surgery

Liver resection

Cardiac surgery

Emergent surgery (any type)

Surgery with high anticipated blood loss

which was significantly higher than that in cirrhotic patients undergoing elective surgical procedures.[39]

Abdominal surgical procedures, including cholecystectomy, gastric bypass, biliary procedures, ulcer surgery, and colonic resection, result in an increased morbidity and mortality in patients with cirrhosis. In a 2007 study by Teh and colleagues,[42] 586 cirrhotic patients underwent major digestive system surgery including esophageal, gastric, intestinal, hepatic, and splenic procedures. The type of procedure did not affect the outcome, but older age and higher MELD score predicted an increased risk of short-term and long-term mortality, with a median survival of almost 5 years for a MELD score of less than 8, but only 14-day median survival if the MELD score was greater than 26.

Three small studies[15,44,45] have evaluated the role of preoperative TIPS insertion in patients with cirrhosis and portal hypertension undergoing extrahepatic abdominal operations. Although the premise of reducing portal hypertension before a major abdominal operation makes sense, the results were mixed, and so no recommendations can be made in support of preoperative TIPS placement.

Cardiac surgery involving cardiopulmonary bypass also carries an increased perioperative risk in patients with cirrhosis. One of the largest studies reviewed 44 cirrhotic patients undergoing either cardiac bypass grafting, valve replacement, or pericardiectomy.[38] Twelve patients developed hepatic decompensation and 7 patients died. The authors concluded that cardiac surgery could be conducted safely if the CTP score was 7 or less. Two additional studies[46,47] confirmed the results of the aforementioned study and support the findings that Child's class is an accurate predictor of hepatic decompensation and mortality following cardiac surgery. Mortality tends to be related to gastrointestinal complications, hemorrhage, and sepsis, as opposed to cardiac failure. Thus, whenever possible, major cardiac operations should be avoided in patients with cirrhosis and the least invasive means of treating coronary disease should be sought.[48]

Patients sustaining trauma who are found to have cirrhosis at the time of laparotomy are at an increased risk of morbidity and mortality following surgery. In one study, 40 cirrhotic patients undergoing laparotomy following trauma had a significantly higher mortality of 45% versus 24% in matched noncirrhotic controls. The increased morbidity and mortality was even true in cirrhotic patients who suffered minor trauma.[49]

Surgical resection in patients with liver disease raises concerns about the adequacy of residual hepatic mass in patients who have compromised function to begin with. Most patients with hepatocellular carcinoma have significant underlying liver disease, and so it is not surprising therefore that such patients have high rates of postsurgical complications, hepatic decompensation, and death.[50] Although cirrhosis is no longer considered a contraindication to hepatic resection, morbidity and mortality are still substantial, with mortality rates quoted as high as 16% and morbidity as high as 60%.[51–57] The improvement in outcomes over the years is likely multifactorial, related to better patient selection, improved intra- and postoperative monitoring, and advancements in surgical techniques.[58,59]

ANESTHESIA

Liver disease can significantly impair the metabolism of anesthetics and certain medications used during surgery. Hepatic dysfunction can affect the distribution, metabolism, and excretion of drugs. Caution must be taken in deciding which drugs to use.

The clinician should also be mindful of the class of drugs, drug doses, and scheduling when confronting postoperative decompensation.

Of the volatile anesthetics, isoflurane is generally recommended as it undergoes the least amount of hepatic metabolism and does not affect hepatic blood flow.[60] Halothane, in contrast, undergoes significant hepatic metabolism and reduces hepatic blood flow. Halothane is a known culprit of severe hepatic injury and has been reported to be the cause of acute liver failure.[61,62] The incidence of acute liver failure is approximately 1 case in 6,000 to 35,000 patients after exposure.[63] This concern has all but eliminated the use of halothane in the United States.

Hepatic dysfunction can result in a longer half-life of many drugs as a result of impairment of the cytochrome P450 enzymes. The perioperative use of certain narcotic opioids, such as morphine and oxycodone, should be avoided in patients with cirrhosis or significant hepatic impairment. The bioavailability of such drugs is markedly increased and their half-life prolonged.[64] Fentanyl, however, does not seem to be affected by hepatic dysfunction.[65]

The metabolism of certain benzodiazepines such as diazepam and midazolam may be slowed in patients with cirrhosis and impaired liver function. Because of their ability to undergo conjugation without hepatic metabolism, benzodiazepines such as oxazepam and temazepam are not affected.[66–68] The increased duration of action of benzodiazepines and narcotics in patients with cirrhosis and liver dysfunction can lead to prolonged depression of the central nervous system and may act as precipitants of hepatic encephalopathy.

Anesthesia can lead to changes in blood flow to the liver that can occur with general or regional anesthesia, meaning the risk of decompensation after surgery is not reduced even if local or spinal anesthesia is used.[60,69] Advanced liver disease is typically associated with systemic and splanchnic vasodilation that leads to activation of the sympathetic nervous system in an attempt to maintain arterial perfusion.[70] The normal cardiac inotropic and chronotropic response to stress may be decreased in cirrhotic patients,[71] and the combination of a hyperdynamic circulation without compensatory mechanisms can lead to hepatic hypoperfusion during surgery. This can be exacerbated by the type of surgery (particularly laparotomy or cardiac surgery), hemorrhage, vasoactive medications, and even patient positioning.[72]

SUMMARY

Preexisting liver disease can lead to significant mortality after surgery. The severity of liver disease measured by the CTP score and the MELD score are relatively accurate predictors of outcome after surgery but are influenced by the type of surgery and the urgency. The algorithms shown in **Figs. 1** and **2** summarize our recommendations using the available literature. In general, Child's class A or MELD score less than 10 are at low risk for death after elective surgery; Child's B or MELD 10 to 15 are at moderate risk, and surgery should be considered depending on the indication and urgency; Child's C or MELD greater than 15 are at high risk, and surgery should be avoided or deferred until the clinical situation changes.

REFERENCES

1. Garrison RN, Cryer HM, Howard DA, et al. Clarification of risk factors for abdominal operations in patients with hepatic cirrhosis. Ann Surg 1984;199(6):648–55.
2. Schemel WH. Unexpected hepatic dysfunction found by multiple laboratory screening. Anesth Analg 1976;55(6):810–2.

3. Hay JE, Czaja AJ, Rakela J, et al. The nature of unexplained chronic aminotransferase elevations of a mild to moderate degree in asymptomatic patients. Hepatology 1989;9(2):193–7.

4. Hultcrantz R, Glaumann H, Lindberg G, et al. Liver investigation in 149 asymptomatic patients with moderately elevated activities of serum aminotransferases. Scand J Gastroenterol 1986;21(1):109–13.

5. Friedman LS, Maddrey WC. Surgery in the patient with liver disease. Med Clin North Am 1987;71(3):453–76.

6. Friedman LS. The risk of surgery in patients with liver disease. Hepatology 1999; 29(6):1617–23.

7. Patel T. Surgery in the patient with liver disease. Mayo Clin Proc 1999;74(6):593–9.

8. Harville DD, Summerskill WH. Sugery in acute hepatitis. Causes and effects. JAMA 1963;27(184):257–61.

9. Powell-Jackson P, Greenway B, Williams R. Adverse effects of exploratory laparotomy in patients with unsuspected liver disease. Br J Surg 1982;69(8):449–51.

10. Greenwood SM, Leffler CT, Minkowitz S. The increased mortality rate of open liver biopsy in alcoholic hepatitis. Surg Gynecol Obstet 1972;134(4):600–4.

11. Higashi H, Matsumata T, Adachi E, et al. Influence of viral hepatitis status on operative morbidity and mortality in patients with primary hepatocellular carcinoma. Br J Surg 1994;81(9):1342–5.

12. Hargrove MD Jr. Chronic active hepatitis: Possible adverse effect of exploratory laparotomy. Surgery 1970;68(5):771–3.

13. Ko S, Nakajima Y, Kanehiro H, et al. Influence of associated viral hepatitis status on recurrence of hepatocellular carcinoma after hepatectomy. World J Surg 1996; 20(8):1082–6.

14. Bruix J, Castells A, Bosch J, et al. Surgical resection of hepatocellular carcinoma in cirrhotic patients: prognostic value of preoperative portal pressure. Gastroenterology 1996;111(4):1018–22.

15. Azoulay D, Buabse F, Damiano I, et al. Neoadjuvant transjugular intrahepatic portosystemic shunt: a solution for extrahepatic abdominal operation in cirrhotic patients with severe portal hypertension. J Am Coll Surg 2001;193(1):46–51.

16. Behrns KE, Tsiotos GG, DeSouza NF, et al. Hepatic steatosis as a potential risk factor for major hepatic resection. J Gastrointest Surg 1998;2(3):292–8.

17. Brolin RE, Bradley LJ, Taliwal RV, et al. Unsuspected cirrhosis discovered during elective obesity operations. Arch Surg 1998;133(1):84–8.

18. Dixon JM, Armstrong CP, Duffy SW, et al. Factors affecting morbidity and mortality after surgery for obstructive jaundice: a review of 373 patients. Gut 1983;24(9):845–52.

19. Greig JD, Krukowski ZH, Matheson NA. Surgical morbidity and mortality in one hundred and twenty-nine patients with obstructive jaundice. Br J Surg 1988; 75(3):216–9.

20. Shirahatti RG, Alphonso N, Joshi RM, et al. Palliative surgery in malignant obstructive jaundice: prognostic indicators of early mortality. J R Coll Surg Edinb 1997;42(4):238–43.

21. Hatfield AR, Tobias R, Terblanche J, et al. Preoperative external biliary drainage in obstructive jaundice. A prospective control trial. Lancet 1982;2(8304):896–9.

22. McPherson GA, Benjamin IS, Hodgson HJ, et al. Pre-operative percutaneous transhepatic biliary drainage: the results of a controlled trial. Br J Surg 1984; 71(5):371–5.

23. Pitt HA, Gomes AS, Mann LL, et al. Does preoperative percutaneous biliary drainage reduce operative risk or increase hospital cost? Ann Surg 1985; 201(5):545–53.

24. Clements WD, Diamond T, McCrory DC, et al. Biliary drainage in obstructive jaundice: experimental and clinical aspects. Br J Surg 1993;80(7):834–42.
25. Lai EC, Mok FP, Fan ST, et al. Preoperative endoscopic drainage for malignant obstructive jaundice. Br J Surg 1994;81(8):1195–8.
26. Child CG, Turcotte JG. Surgery and portal hypertension. Major Probl Clin Surg 1964;1:1–85.
27. Pugh RN, Murray-Lyon IM, Dawson JL. Transection of the oesophagus for bleeding oesophageal varices. Br J Surg 1973;60(8):646–9.
28. Mansour A, Watson W, Shayani V, et al. Abdominal operations in patients with cirrhosis: still a major surgical challenge. Surgery 1997;122(4):730–5.
29. Ziser A, Plevak DJ, Wiesner RH, et al. Morbidity and mortality in cirrhotic patients undergoing anesthesia and surgery. Anesthesiology 1999;90(1):42–53.
30. Malinchoc M, Kamath PS, Gordon FD, et al. A model to predict poor survival in patients undergoing transjugular intrahepatic portosystemic shunts. Hepatology 2000;31(4):864–71.
31. Said A, Williams J, Holden J, et al. Model for end stage liver disease score predicts mortality across a broad spectrum of liver disease. J Hepatol 2004; 40(6):897–903.
32. Chalasani N, Kahi C, Francois F, et al. Model for end-stage liver disease (MELD) for predicting mortality in patients with acute variceal bleeding. Hepatology 2002; 35(5):1282–4.
33. Ben-Ari Z, Cardin F, McCormick AP, et al. A predictive model for failure to control bleeding during acute variceal haemorrhage. J Hepatol 1999;31(3):443–50.
34. Sheth M, Riggs M, Patel T. Utility of the Mayo End-Stage Liver Disease (MELD) score in assessing prognosis of patients with alcoholic hepatitis. BMC Gastroenterol 2002;2:2.
35. Yantorno SE, Kremers WK, Ruf AE, et al. MELD is superior to King's college and Clichy's criteria to assess prognosis in fulminant hepatic failure. Liver Transpl 2007;13(6):822–8.
36. Schmidt LE, Larsen FS. MELD score as a predictor of liver failure and death in patients with acetaminophen induced liver injury. Hepatology 2007;45(3):789–96.
37. Perkins L, Jeffries M, Patel T. Utility of preoperative scores for predicting morbidity after cholecystectomy in patients with cirrhosis. Clin Gastroenterol Hepatol 2004;2(12):1123–8.
38. Suman A, Barnes DS, Zein NN, et al. Predicting outcome after cardiac surgery in patients with cirrhosis: a comparison of Child-Pugh and MELD scores. Clin Gastroenterol Hepatol 2004;2(8):719–23.
39. Farnsworth N, Fagan SP, Berger DH, et al. Child-Turcotte-Pugh versus MELD score as a predictor of outcome after elective and emergent surgery in cirrhotic patients. Am J Surg 2004;188(5):580–3.
40. Befeler AS, Palmer DE, Hoffman M, et al. The safety of intra-abdominal surgery in patients with cirrhosis: model for end stage liver disease score is superior to Child-Turcotte-Pugh classification in predicting outcome. Arch Surg 2005; 140(7):650–4.
41. Cucchetti A, Ercolani G, Vivarelli M, et al. Impact of model for end-stage liver disease (MELD) score on prognosis after hepatectomy for hepatocellular carcinoma on cirrhosis. Liver Transpl 2006;12(6):966–71.
42. Teh SH, Nagorney DM, Stevens SR, et al. Risk factors for mortality after surgery in patients with cirrhosis. Gastroenterology 2007;132(4):1609–11.
43. Hanje AJ, Patel T. Preoperative evaluation of patients with liver disease. Nat Clin Pract Gastroenterol Hepatol 2007;4(5):266–76.

44. Gil A, Martinez-Regueira F, Hernandez-Lizoain JL, et al. The role of transjugular intrahepatic portosystemic shunt prior to abdominal tumoral surgery in cirrhotic patients with portal hypertension. Eur J Surg Oncol 2004;30(1):46–52.
45. Vinet E, Perreault P, Bouchard L, et al. Transjugular intrahepatic portosystemic shunt before abdominal surgery in cirrhotic patients: a retrospective, comparative study. Can J Gastroenterol 2006;20(6):401–4.
46. Klemperer JD, Ko W, Krieger KH, et al. Cardiac operation in patients with cirrhosis. Ann Thorac Surg 1998;65(1):85–7.
47. Filsoufi F, Salzberg SP, Rahmanian PB, et al. Early and late outcome of cardiac surgery in patients with liver cirrhosis. Liver Transpl 2007;13(7):990–5.
48. Gaudino M, Santarelli P, Bruno P, et al. Palliative coronary artery surgery in patients with severe noncardiac diseases. Am J Cardiol 1997;80(10):1351–2.
49. Demetriades D, Constantinou C, Salim A, et al. Liver cirrhosis in patients undergoing laparotomy for trauma: effect on outcomes. J Am Coll Surg 2004;199(4):538–42.
50. Clavien PA, Petrowsky H, DeOliveira ML, et al. Strategies for safer liver surgery and partial liver transplantation. N Engl J Med 2007;356(15):1545–59.
51. MacIntosh EL, Minuk GY. Hepatic resection in patients with cirrhosis and hepatocellular carcinoma. Surg Gynecol Obstet 1992;174(3):245–54.
52. Wu CC, Ho WL, Yeh DC, et al. Hepatic resection of hepatocellular carcinoma in cirrhotic livers: is it unjustified in impaired liver function? Surgery 1996;120(1):34–9.
53. Bruix J. Treatment of hepatocellular carcinoma. Hepatology 1996;25(2):259–62.
54. Cohnert TU, Rau HG, Buttler E, et al. Preoperative risk assessment of hepatic resection for malignancy disease. World J Surg 1997;21(4):396–400.
55. Capussotti L, Polastri R. Operative risks of major hepatic resections. Hepatogastroenterology 1998;45(19):184–90.
56. Mor E, Kaspa RT, Sheiner P, et al. Treatment of hepatocellular carcinoma associated with cirrhosis in the era of liver transplantation. Ann Intern Med 1998;129(8):643–53.
57. Di Bisceglie AM, Carither RL Jr, Gores GJ. Hepatocellular carcinoma. Hepatology 1998;28(4):1161–5.
58. Wu CC, Yeh DC, Lin MC, et al. Improving operative safety for cirrhotic liver resection. Br J Surg 2001;88(2):210–5.
59. Grazi GL, Ercolani G, Pierangeli F, et al. Improved results of liver resection for hepatocellular carcinoma give the procedure added value. Ann Surg 2001;234(1):71–8.
60. Gelman S, Fowler KC, Smith LR. Liver circulation and function during isoflurane and halothane anesthesia. Anesthesiology 1984;61(6):726–30.
61. Kenna JG. Immunoallergic drug-induced hepatitis: lessons from halothane. J Hepatol 1997;26(1):5–12.
62. Daghfous R, el Aidli S, Sfaxi M, et al. Halothane-induced hepatitis: 8 case reports. Tunis Med 2003;81(11):874–8.
63. Gut J. Molecular basis of halothane hepatitis. Arch Toxicol Suppl 1998;20:3–17.
64. Delco F, Tchambaz L, Schlienger R, et al. Dose adjustment in patients with liver disease. Drug Saf 2005;28(6):529–45.
65. Tegeder I, Lotsch J, Geisslinger G. Pharmacokinetics of opioids in liver disease. Clin Pharmacokinet 1999;37(1):17–40.
66. Ochs HR, Greenblatt DJ, Eckardt B, et al. Repeated diazepam dosing in cirrhotic patients: cumulation and sedation. Clin Pharmacol Ther 1983;33(4):471–6.
67. Ghabrial H, Desmond PV, Watson KJ, et al. The effects of age and chronic liver disease on the elimination of temazepam. Eur J Clin Pharmacol 1986;30(1):93–7.

68. Pentikainen PJ, Valisalmi L, Himberg JJ, et al. Pharmacokinetics of midazolam following intravenous and oral administration in patients with chronic liver disease and in healthy subjects. J Clin Pharmacol 1989;29(3):272–7.
69. Darling JR, Murray JM, Hainsworth AM, et al. The effect of isoflurane or spinal anesthesia on indocyanine green disappearance rate in the elderly. Anesth Analg 1994;78(4):706–9.
70. Groszmann RJ. Hyperdynamic circulation of liver disease 40 years later: pathophysiology and clinical consequences. Hepatology 1994;20(5):1359–63.
71. Moller S, Henriksen JH. Cirrhotic cardiomyopathy: a pathophysiological review of circulatory dysfunction in liver disease. Heart 2002;87(1):9–15.
72. Gelman SI. Disturbances in hepatic blood flow during anesthesia and surgery. Arch Surg 1976;111(8):881–3.

Liver Transplantation: From Child to MELD

Juan F. Gallegos-Orozco, MD[a], Hugo E. Vargas, MD[b],*

KEYWORDS

- Cirrhosis • Liver disease • Viral hepatitis
- Hepatocellular carcinoma • Liver transplantation

Since the first successful liver transplant by Dr. Thomas Starzl in 1967, the procedure has become an established treatment for patients with end-stage liver disease (ESLD) of any cause. A combination of advances in surgical technique, patient selection, improved perioperative care, and availability of adequate immunosuppressive agents, has resulted in a significant improvement in overall patient survival after transplantation. Current data from the Organ Procurement and Transplantation Network (OPTN) in the United States reveals 1-, 3-, and 5-year patient survival of 87%, 79%, and 73%, respectively (UNOS/OPTN, www.optn.org, accessed November, 2008). Similar results are reported from Europe, with 82%, 75%, and 71% recipients alive at 1, 3, and 5 years after transplantation in more than 65,000 surgeries since 1988 (www.eltr.org, accessed November, 2008).

The widespread availability of transplantation in most major medical centers in the United States, together with a growing number of transplant candidates, has made it necessary for primary care providers, especially Internal Medicine and Family Practice physicians to be active in the clinical care of these patients before and after transplantation. This review provides an overview of the liver transplantation process, including indications, contraindications, time of referral to a transplant center, and the current organ allocation system, and briefly touches on the expanding field of living donor liver transplantation (LDLT).

INDICATIONS FOR LIVER TRANSPLANTATION IN CIRRHOSIS

Liver transplantation is the current standard therapy for patients with acute or chronic irreversible liver failure, for selected metabolic derangements without liver failure (primary oxaluria, familial amyloid polyneuropathy), and malignant disease confined

[a] Division of Gastroenterology, Department of Medicine, Mayo Clinic Arizona, 13400 E. Shea Boulevard, Scottsdale, AZ 85259, USA
[b] Division of Transplantation Medicine, Department of Medicine, Mayo Clinic Arizona, 5777 E. Mayo Boulevard, Phoenix, AZ 85054, USA
* Corresponding author.
E-mail address: vargas.hugo@mayo.edu (H.E. Vargas).

Med Clin N Am 93 (2009) 931–950
doi:10.1016/j.mcna.2009.03.010
0025-7125/09/$ – see front matter © 2009 Elsevier Inc. All rights reserved.

medical.theclinics.com

to the liver. The main objectives of liver transplantation are to improve patient survival, functional status, and quality of life.[1,2]

The leading indications for liver transplantation in the United States and Europe are hepatitis C and cirrhosis induced by alcoholic liver disease. In 2007, 6493 liver transplants were performed in the United States. The main causes were hepatitis C (26.5%), followed by hepatocellular carcinoma (HCC, with or without cirrhosis, 14%), alcoholic liver disease (10%), primary biliary cirrhosis (PBC), primary sclerosing cholangitis (PSC, 8%), cryptogenic cirrhosis (5.5%), and nonalcoholic steatohepatitis (4.5%) (UNOS/OPTN, www.optn.org/latestData/rptData.asp, accessed November 2008).

SELECTED INDICATIONS
Chronic Hepatitis C

Cirrhosis from chronic hepatitis C is the main indication for liver transplantation in the United States. It is estimated that the number of patients with cirrhosis from HCV infection will increase in the next few decades,[3] and will certainly result in a greater number of cases of ESLD and HCC, hence increasing the number of liver transplants related to HCV.[4–7] At present, up to 20% of subjects with chronic hepatitis C go on to develop cirrhosis,[8] and once this occurs, they have a 2% to 8% annual risk of developing HCC.[9] The 10-year survival for patients with compensated HCV cirrhosis is greater than 80%, but is significantly reduced to less than 50% at 5 years once any of the complications of liver cirrhosis develop, making these patients candidates for liver transplantation.[10]

Post-transplant HCV viremia and graft infection is the rule. Disease progression in these patients is accelerated compared with the nontransplant population.[11] Recent series have documented a significant decrease in long-term survival after liver transplantation in HCV recipients compared with other causes of ESLD.[12–14]

Antiviral therapy for HCV patients in the pre- and post-transplant period is complex and should only be carried out by experienced clinicians in transplant centers. If patients are able to clear the virus before transplantation, they have a better outcome than nonresponders.[15] Some groups have had success treating liver transplant recipients after they have developed a significant histologic recurrence of HCV.[4,7,16–19] Even so, HCV will continue to pose significant challenges to the transplant community in years to come.

Alcoholic Cirrhosis

Alcoholic liver disease (ALD) is one of the most frequent causes of cirrhosis in the United States and Europe, and hence is often encountered in the transplant population. Abstinence from alcohol has a positive effect on patients with ALD and even patients with decompensated cirrhosis may derive a survival benefit and be able to delay or even avoid transplantation altogether.[20,21]

Patients with ALD being considered for transplantation are at risk of post-transplant recidivism and most centers require a minimum of 6 months of demonstrated abstinence and an adequate evaluation and treatment period for alcohol addiction, before considering a candidate for transplant.[22] A varying number of recipients will relapse after transplantation, but graft loss secondary to severe recidivism is infrequent.[23–25]

Once transplanted, the survival for these patients is similar to that observed for other conditions, with 7-year survival rates of 60%.[26–29] Physicians taking care of these patients after transplantation should be aware that they have an increased risk of developing head and neck, esophageal, and gastric malignancies.[30,31]

Primary Biliary Cirrhosis and Primary Sclerosing Cholangitis

PBC and PSC are chronic inflammatory and destructive cholestatic disorders that lead to ESLD. The only effective treatment in such patients is liver transplantation, which results in excellent survival, with 1-year and 5-year survival rates of 90% and 82%, respectively.[32]

Selected patients with severe pruritus and impaired quality of life from PBC are candidates for transplantation, even in the presence of preserved liver function.[33,34] Recurrence of PBC after transplantation has been well documented, but does not have a significant impact on patient and graft survival.[35]

Patients with PSC also do well after transplantation,[36–39] although recent data demonstrated increased retransplantation rates and decreased survival compared with other indications, including PBC.[40,41]

Patients with PSC are at high risk of developing cholangiocarcinoma and every effort should be taken to reasonably exclude the diagnosis before transplantation, as its presence has a significant negative impact on postoperative survival.[38] After transplantation, patients with PSC and ulcerative colitis should undergo regular surveillance by colonoscopy to detect colorectal cancer, as this can adversely affect post-transplant survival.[39,42,43]

Hepatocellular Carcinoma

HCC, the most frequent primary liver malignancy, is a worldwide health problem responsible for close to 1 million deaths each year.[10] Most cases are related to chronic hepatitis B virus infection, but a significant increase has been noted in Western countries as a direct consequence of chronic hepatitis C.[44–46] Prognosis in these patients is related to tumor stage and liver function.[47–49]

A wide variety of surgical and nonsurgical therapies are available, but for selected patients with decompensated cirrhosis and malignancy confined to the liver, the best outcomes have been obtained with liver transplantation. In 2007, almost 15% of all liver transplants in the United States were related to HCC (UNOS/OPTN, www.optn.org, accessed November, 2008). The 5-year survival for patients transplanted for malignant neoplasms of the liver in the United States from 2000 to 2005 was 65%, significantly better than the 46% for those who received a liver transplant in the mid-1990s.[32,50] The key for improved survival is adequate patient selection, and the best outcomes have been obtained in patients with stage I and II HCC as assessed by the tumor-node-metastasis (TNM) staging classification. Essentially, patient selection is limited to cases with a single nodule less than or equal to 1.9 cm (stage I) or a single nodule 2 to 5 cm in diameter or 2 to 3 nodules all less than 3 cm each (stage II) (Liver allocation policy UNOS June 2008 at www.unos.org, accessed November 2008).[51]

CONTRAINDICATIONS TO LIVER TRANSPLANTATION IN CIRRHOSIS

To accomplish the goals of increasing survival and improving quality of life, liver transplant candidates must be sick enough to require an organ transplant, but not so sick that they would be unable to withstand the procedure or that the transplant itself would increase their morbidity or shorten their survival. All potential candidates should undergo an extensive medical evaluation to exclude those that will be harmed by the procedure.

Refinements in surgical technique and improved medical care of the transplant patient have resulted in an increase in the number of indications for transplantation and a decrease in absolute and relative contraindications (**Box 1**).[1,52,53]

Box 1
Absolute contraindications to liver transplantation

Active substance abuse

Inadequate social support, extreme psychosocial dysfunction, active psychosis or other underlying psychosocial pathology severely hampering compliance with peritransplant care and postoperative management

Unstable, active cardiopulmonary disease

  Symptomatic ischemic heart disease

  Severe pulmonary hypertension

Active, incurable extrahepatic malignancy

  Nonhepatic malignancy

  Hepatocellular carcinoma with capsular invasion or distant metastases

  Cholangiocarcinoma with extension to adjacent nonhepatic tissues

Active, uncontrolled and untreatable sepsis

Active HIV infection, AIDS-defining illness or HIV unresponsive to highly active antiretroviral therapy

Anatomic anomaly or extensive vascular thromboses precluding transplantation

Data from Everson GT, Membreno FE. Liver transplantation: indication, contraindications and results. In: Rodés J, Benhamou JP, Blei A, et al, editors. Textbook of hepatology: from basic science to clinical practice. 3rd edition. Oxford: Blackwell Publishing; 2007. p. 1984–95.

Most transplant centers have their own set of exclusion criteria or contraindications to transplantation, but they can be divided into psychosocial, medical, and technical criteria.

Psychosocial

All potential candidates should be expected to comply with medical care after transplantation and demonstrate an adequate social and family support system, to increase the success rate of the procedure. Patients should not be listed for transplantation unless these expectations are reasonably satisfied.

Active alcohol and substance abuse, including tobacco abuse in some centers, are deemed absolute contraindications to transplantation.[10] Patients with past addictive behaviors should undergo psychological or psychiatric counseling and be able to document a minimum of 3 to 6 months of abstinence from alcohol, illicit drugs, and, in some institutions, from tobacco. Most centers perform random serum and urine drug screening tests to ensure compliance with recommendations. Patients are made aware that documented relapse may jeopardize their transplant candidacy.

Medical Contraindications

Age

There is no specific age limit for transplantation, as long as the candidate is deemed well enough to undergo the procedure, but most centers in general avoid transplanting patients older than 65 years, as there seems to be a decreased survival rate in this age group compared with younger recipients.[53,54]

Cardiovascular disease

In the United States there is an ever-growing problem with cardiovascular disease, hence transplant candidates frequently have a history of cardiovascular disease. Underlying coronary artery disease (CAD) is present in 2.5% to 27% of liver transplant candidates.[55,56] Patients with active CAD, severe systolic dysfunction, advanced cardiomyopathy, severe pulmonary hypertension, and severe valvular heart disease, should not undergo liver transplantation.[10,57,58] A comprehensive cardiovascular evaluation should be performed in patients at high risk, such as those older than 50 years, active smokers, and diabetics, according to the policies of each transplant center.[10,53]

Pulmonary disease

Absolute pulmonary contraindications to liver transplantation include severe or oxygen-dependent chronic obstructive pulmonary disease and advanced pulmonary fibrosis, and the presence of severe pulmonary hypertension (mean pulmonary artery pressure ≥50 mm Hg). Asthma, hepatic hydrothorax, and pulmonary infections are amenable to adequate medical therapy before transplantation and, hence, should be considered only relative contraindications.[1] Patients with active pulmonary tuberculosis should receive adequate treatment before transplantation and remain on therapy 1 year after surgery.[1]

Cirrhotic patients are at risk of developing 2 distinct pulmonary entities: hepatopulmonary syndrome (HPS) and portopulmonary hypertension.

HPS is a triad of chronic end-stage liver disease, arterial deoxygenation, and diffuse intrapulmonary vasodilation that is present in 1% to 2% of cirrhotic patients.[52,59,60] In recent years HPS has been accepted as an indication for liver transplantation in selected cases; however patients with severe hypoxia have significantly increased perioperative mortality.[10,60–62] Recent guidelines from the American Association for the Study of Liver Diseases (AASLD) recommend that cirrhotic patients with severe HPS undergo expedited referral and transplant evaluation to improve their extremely poor prognosis.[10]

Portopulmonary hypertension is present in 2% to 4% of patients with advanced cirrhosis.[60,63] Mild and moderate pulmonary hypertension does not preclude liver transplant. New modalities (oral, inhaled, and injectable) have been introduced in recent years to decrease pulmonary pressures and allow a "surgical window" for liver transplantation.[64] However, uncontrolled severe portopulmonary hypertension is an absolute contraindication to transplantation.[10,60,65]

Kidney disease

The presence of acute or chronic kidney disease does not constitute an absolute contraindication to liver transplantation, but has been demonstrated to be a risk factor for poor postoperative outcomes. Specifically, patients with pre-existing kidney disease have an increased rate of postoperative dialysis and decreased long-term survival after liver transplant.[52,66,67] In patients with chronic kidney disease who also develop end-stage liver disease, consideration should be given to the possibility of a combined kidney-liver transplant.[10]

Hepatorenal syndrome (HRS), notably the rapidly progressive HRS (type 1), is specific to patients with advanced cirrhosis and ascites, and generally has an ominous prognosis. Liver transplantation in such cases has been shown to revert renal failure and improve survival,[68,69] hence expedited referral and evaluation for liver transplantation is currently recommended.[10] Vasoactive agents such as terlipressin will play a role in preventing early dialysis and death in liver transplant candidates with this complication.[70,71]

Obesity

Liver transplant candidates are frequently overweight or obese, and certainly this trend will increase in the United Sates, as the obesity epidemic continues. Unfortunately, liver transplant recipients with obesity, defined by a body mass index (BMI) >35 kg/m^2, have significantly reduced 5-year survival compared with nonobese patients.[72] This is more significant in patients with morbid obesity (BMI >40 kg/m^2), as they suffer from increased rates of primary nonfunction and decreased rates of 30-day, 1- and 2-year post-transplantation survival.[72] From these data, the current AASLD guidelines recommend that morbid obesity be considered an absolute contraindication to transplantation.[10]

Diabetes mellitus

Up to 15% of transplant candidates have diabetes mellitus (predominantly type 2).[52] Patients should have adequate metabolic control before proceeding with liver transplantation and be free of significant comorbidities from the diabetes. Recent data have suggested that diabetic recipients do not have as good outcomes as nondiabetic patients, with 1- and 5-year survival of 67.5% and 61% for diabetics compared with 90% and 77% for nondiabetic recipients. Causes of death in the diabetic population were mostly related to CAD, cerebrovascular disease, and sepsis.[73,74]

Infectious disease

Active pneumonia and uncontrolled sepsis are absolute contraindications to liver transplantation. Other infections, such as bacteremia, osteomyelitis, fungal infections, and pyogenic abscesses, should be aggressively treated before transplantation. Specifically, patients with spontaneous bacterial peritonitis should receive at least 48 hours of antibiotic therapy and have documented eradication of the infection before transplantation.[1,10]

The advent of highly active antiretroviral therapy (HAART) has significantly changed the natural history of HIV infection and the acquired immunodeficiency syndrome (AIDS). As a result, subjects infected by HIV are currently living longer and developing a different set of comorbidities. In recent years, chronic hepatitis C and cirrhosis have emerged as leading causes of death among this patient population. Hence, some transplant centers in the United States and Europe are proceeding with liver transplantation in selected patients with HIV. Their short- and medium-term results are similar to non-HIV patients transplanted for similar indications.[75–77] Even so, most centers in the United States consider infection with HIV to be an absolute contraindication to the procedure,[78] and results of prospective studies are eagerly awaited.

Malignancies

Active extrahepatic malignancy, other than nonmelanoma skin cancer and selected metastatic neuroendocrine tumors, should constitute an absolute contraindication to transplantation. In general, transplanted patients are at increased risk of recurrence mainly due to immunosuppression. There are no specific guidelines for liver transplantation in patients with prior hematologic or solid-organ malignancies, but it is generally accepted that patients be cured for at least 2 years before the procedure. In some specific malignancies, such as melanoma, breast and colon cancer, the disease-free period should probably be further extended to a minimum of 5 years.[1,10]

Surgical and Technical Issues

Current refinements in surgical technique and advances in imaging studies have resulted in a short list of surgical or technical contraindications to transplantation. Portal vein thrombosis is not considered an absolute contraindication, but still confers a poor prognosis for postoperative graft dysfunction and perioperative mortality, especially if the entire portal venous system is occluded or atrophied.[79,80] As part of the pretransplant evaluation process, all patients should be submitted to CT or MRI angiography to adequately assess portal vein system patency, and evaluate for hepatic artery anatomic variants that could result in technically challenging vascular anastomoses.[52]

TIMING OF TRANSPLANTATION REFERRAL

Regardless of the cause, patients with liver cirrhosis who have suffered a clinical decompensation of the disease, namely, hepatic encephalopathy, ascites, spontaneous bacterial peritonitis, or HRS, and HCC, should be considered potential transplantation candidates, as this is the only therapy currently available that will provide significant long-term benefit in patients with an otherwise dismal prognosis.[52,53] Patients who develop any of these complications have a significantly increased risk of mortality compared with cirrhotic patients with compensated disease.[81]

As most patients with cirrhosis are cared for by primary care providers, practitioners should be aware of not only the general indications for liver transplantation but also of the best timing for referral to a transplant center. In general, early referral is better than late referral, as this gives the transplant center time to adequately assess a patient's candidacy for transplantation, and provide expertise in the medical management of patients with complications from cirrhosis. A close professional relationship should be established between the transplant center and the referring physician to improve overall patient care in the pre- and post-transplant setting.

As a general rule, liver transplantation should be offered to patients in whom survival without the procedure would be worse than with the intervention, and after all available medical therapies have proved ineffective.[82] Recent recommendations from American and European consensus conferences of liver transplant experts have been published and provide helpful clinical guidelines for physicians involved in the care of the transplant patient.[10,83,84] Specifically, the AASLD in the United States has recommended that patients with cirrhosis be referred to a transplant center when they develop evidence of hepatic dysfunction based on a Child-Turcotte-Pugh score more than or equal to 7 (**Table 1**) or a Model for End-stage Liver Disease (MELD) score more than or equal to 10; or when they experience their first major complication (ascites, variceal bleeding, or hepatic encephalopathy). Referral is also indicated in selected

Table 1
Child-Pugh-Turcotte scoring system to assess liver disease severity

Variable	1 Point	2 Points	3 Points
Encephalopathy	None	Grade 1–2	Grade 3–4
Ascites	Absent	Slight	Moderate
Bilirubin (mg/dL)	1–2	2–3	>3
For PBC	1–4	4–10	>10
Albumin (g/dL)	>3.5	2.8–3.5	<2.8
Prothrombin time (seconds prolonged)	1–4	4–6	>6
Or INR	<1.7	1.7–2.3	>2.3

Class A (5–6 points); class B (7–9 points); class C ($\geq$ 10 points).
Abbreviations: PBC, primary biliary cirrhosis; INR, international normalized ratio of prothrombin time.

subjects in the absence of the above criteria, for example, in patients with early HCC or with PBC and significantly impaired quality of life.[10]

OVERVIEW OF THE PRETRANSPLANT EVALUATION PROCESS

Once a patient has been referred for consideration of liver transplantation, the transplant center should perform a timely and thorough evaluation to address the following issues[10]:

1. Can the patient survive the operation and the immediate postoperative period?
2. Can the patient be expected to comply with the complex medical regimen required after liver transplantation?
3. Does the patient have other comorbid conditions that could so severely compromise graft or patient survival that transplantation would be futile and an inappropriate use of a scarce donor organ?

Most transplant centers perform a multidisciplinary evaluation, which commonly includes a careful history and physical examination by a transplant hepatologist, and visits with a transplant surgeon, psychologist or psychiatrist, infectious diseases specialist, transplant coordinator, social worker, and a finances counselor. In selected cases, patients may undergo further evaluation from other specialists such as cardiologists, oncologists, and pulmonary medicine specialists, as well as further counseling in cases with a history of alcohol or drug abuse.

Laboratory tests are obtained to (1) confirm the cause of liver disease (serologies for viral hepatitis B and C, autoimmune hepatitis, hemochromatosis, Wilson disease, α-1 antitrypsin deficiency); (2) assess liver function (aminotransferases, bilirubin, alkaline phosphatase, total protein, albumin, international normalized ratio of prothrombin time [INR]); (3) document the status of relevant past or present infections (cytomegalovirus, Epstein-Barr virus, HIV, syphilis); (4) evaluate renal function (blood urea nitrogen [BUN], creatinine, creatinine clearance, cystatin-C); (5) determine blood type for listing purposes; (6) screen for HCC or cholangiocarcinoma (α-fetoprotein, carcinoembryonic antigen [CEA], CA 19-9).[10,85]

Imaging studies are indicated to exclude HCC or define its extent (CT or MRI), and to assess hepatic artery anatomy and portal and hepatic vein patency (Doppler ultrasound, CT or MR angiography). In patients with PSC, imaging studies may include magnetic resonance cholangiopancreatography (MRCP) or endoscopic retrograde cholangiopancreatography (ERCP) with biopsy or brushings in an effort to rule out cholangiocarcinoma before transplantation, as this generally constitutes a contraindication to the procedure.

All candidates undergo a complete cardiopulmonary assessment that includes electrocardiogram, cardiac echocardiography, cardiac stress testing (dobutamine echocardiography or nuclear medicine), chest radiograph and pulmonary function tests. If the results of cardiac stress tests are positive, patients are generally referred to a cardiologist and undergo coronary angiography.[10,86,87] Transplant candidacy is conditional on the ability to correct the underlying CAD by percutaneous coronary intervention or coronary artery bypass grafting.

Patients should also be up to date with regard to age- and gender-appropriate preventive health services, including influenza and pneumococcal vaccinations, bone mineral density, and accepted screening tests for colon, breast, cervical, and prostate cancer. These services are generally provided by the patient's primary care physician. Patients should also undergo a thorough dental evaluation.

Once all the information is available, the case is discussed by a multidisciplinary patient selection committee and a decision to list or not to list the patient is made. A patient may also be deferred for listing, pending the results of further evaluation for specific medical, surgical, or psychosocial issues.

ORGAN ALLOCATION POLICIES: FROM CHILD TO MELD AND BEYOND

As liver transplantation has become the definitive therapy for ESLD, the need for distributing a scarce resource has become critical to the success of the procedure (**Fig. 1**).

Different countries have established there own policies with regard to organ donation, distribution, and allocation to meet their own particular needs. In 1984, the US Federal Government passed the National Organ Transplant Act (NOTA sections 371–376 of the Public Health Service Act, 1984). As a result, the Organ Procurement and Transplantation Network (OPTN) was established in 1986 and has since been operated by the United Network for Organ Sharing (UNOS), a nonprofit organization contracted by the Federal government.[88,89] Their main mission has been to develop policies for organ distribution and allocation, without compromising the ethical principles of medical justice and usefulness.[78] The "allocation to the sickest patient first" policy set forth by the OPTN is in compliance with the Final Rule as designated by the Department of Health and Human Services and privileges medical justice over usefulness.[90]

Child-Turcotte-Pugh Score

In a first effort to classify patients on the transplant waiting list, 4 incremental definitions of disease severity, so-called "status definitions," were created by UNOS: status 1 included all emergency cases; status 2 was established for patients admitted to an ICU; status 3 was for hospitalized patients, and status 4 was used for patients at home. However, it was soon realized that the place of care was not necessarily reflective of the actual severity of the patient's liver disease, and further improvements to the initial allocation system led to the adoption, in 1996, of the Child-Turcotte-Pugh (CTP) scoring system as a measure of disease severity.[88,89] The CTP score is based on clinical and laboratory parameters, namely hepatic encephalopathy, ascites, total bilirubin, prothrombin time, and serum albumin (**Table 1**). Each variable is assigned 1 to 3 points and a final composite score designates patients into 1 of 3 distinct

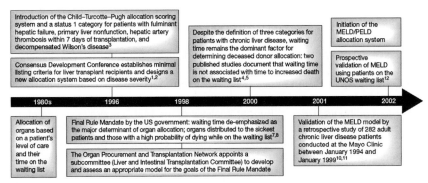

Fig. 1. Timeline of the development of liver allocation policy. (*Adapted from* Wiesner RH. Patient selection in an era of liver donor shortage: current US policy. Nat Clin Pract Gastroenterol Hepatol 2005;2(1):24–30 copyright 2005 Macmillan Publishers Ltd; with permission.)

categories, class A (5–6 points); class B (7–9 points), and class C (10–15 points), that reflect progressive degrees of disease severity.[91] Although originally designed to classify liver disease severity in patients undergoing surgical transection for esophageal varices, it has become a widely applied clinical tool to classify disease severity in patients with chronic liver disease in general.

The addition of the CTP score to the original UNOS classification scheme resulted in a reorganization of status categories for patients with chronic liver disease, such that patients were classified as follows: status 2a (CTP ≥10, admission to the ICU and estimated survival <7 days); status 2b (CTP ≥10 or a CTP ≥7 in patients with 1 or more complications of portal hypertension, and patients with stage 1 and 2 HCC), or status 3 (CTP ≥7), for ambulatory patients who met the minimal listing criteria. Status 1 category was left for patients with fulminant hepatic failure, primary graft nonfunction or hepatic artery thrombosis within 7 days of transplantation, or decompensated Wilson disease, granting them the highest priority on the waiting list.[89]

As the number of patients awaiting a liver transplant grew, each status category became increasingly large and comprised a heterogeneous mix of patients with differing disease severity. By default, candidates were then prioritized by waiting time, as this was the main "tie-breaking" criteria used to allocate an organ within a same status category.[88] Unfortunately, this resulted in significantly disparate waiting times in different transplant centers, as time of listing was more a reflection of time to patient referral and individual transplant center listing policies. Analysis of waiting list mortality did not correlate with waiting list time, suggesting that time on the waiting list was not an adequate parameter to rank transplant candidates.[82] These results, in combination with general dissatisfaction with the limited categorical 4-status system, led the OPTN to seek alternative systems for prioritizing candidates on the waiting list.[88]

MELD Era

It was clear that waiting time on the list needed to be deemphasized, as per the US Government's Final Rule Mandate but also that a new measure of disease severity was needed to replace the CTP score. Even though CTP had been in use for many years and the variables needed to calculate it were readily available, it had several shortcomings. The main shortcoming was the reliance on parameters, such as hepatic encephalopathy, ascites, and prothrombin time, which had poor reproducibility between different transplant centers and laboratories. Another major shortcoming was the "ceiling" effect of the CTP score, such that the maximum score for each parameter is 3 points and thus no difference is made, for example, between a patient with a bilirubin level of 5 mg/dL and a patient with clearly more severe liver dysfunction manifested by a bilirubin level of 20 mg/dL. The other big problem with using CTP score was that it had not been validated as a predictive tool for mortality on the waiting list.

MELD (formerly Mayo end-stage liver disease model) was developed in the late 1990s to assess short-term mortality in patients undergoing transjugular intrahepatic portosystemic shunts (TIPS).[92] Further analysis of the MELD score demonstrated its usefulness as a clinical tool to assess liver disease severity in general[93,94] and it was also found to predict short-term mortality in candidates on the waiting list.[95] This system uses 3 simple biochemical parameters, namely total bilirubin, INR of prothrombin time, and serum creatinine, to assess liver disease severity and can be calculated at www.unos.org/resources/meldPeldCalculator.asp. A similar system has been designed for pediatric patients (Pediatric End-stage Liver Disease [PELD] model).[96]

The MELD score was incorporated into the organ allocation system and implemented by UNOS in February 2002, essentially eliminating waiting time as a significant allocation criterion and using the MELD score as a continuous scale to rank patients with varying liver disease severity.[97] Under this new system, UNOS status 1 has been preserved for emergency cases, and the other categories have been substituted by MELD scores.

Initial assessment of the results of liver transplantation in the United States after implementation of the MELD score for organ allocation revealed that there was a reduction in the number of new patients placed on the waiting list, an increase in the number of procedures performed, and no change in the overall post-transplant survival rate.[98]

A recent evaluation of the MELD scoring system applied to patients on the waiting list revealed that recipients with a score of <15 points actually had greater mortality rate after transplantation then similarly classified patients who remained on the waiting list.[99] This is the basis for the current UNOS "share 15" policy, whereby donor livers are allocated to candidates with MELD >15, within the local or regional organ procurement organization, before offering the organ to local patients with MELD <15.[88,100]

There are specific conditions, such as early HCC, polycystic liver disease, hepatopulmonary syndrome, familial amyloid polyneuropathy, hereditary oxalosis, or hyperammonemia syndromes, for which the MELD scoring system is inadequate for organ prioritization. To deal with these cases, an alternative allocation system based on regional review boards was created. After review of the individual case, the board may assign additional MELD points to the transplant candidates for whom mortality risk is not felt to be adequately assessed by the MELD score.[88,100] Recent guidelines have been published to improve the ability of regional review boards to adequately prioritize such cases.[101]

Several criticisms of MELD have been voiced recently. The biochemical parameters used to calculate the score can be influenced by therapeutic interventions or suffer from significant variations if measured by different techniques or performed by different laboratories.[89] A couple of recent metaanalyses have concluded that the MELD score does not perform better than CTP in assessing prognosis in cases of cirrhosis or in patients on the transplant waiting list.[102,103]

As more data evaluating MELD have been published, it is clear that the predictive ability of the model increases if certain clinical (encephalopathy, ascites) or biochemical (serum sodium) variables are included.[104–107] Further research will certainly result in improvements and fine-tuning of MELD and the allocation system.

The Future

Although the MELD score is useful in assessing the urgency of the recipient, it does not take into account relevant donor variables that have been associated with poor graft outcomes, such as donor age, gender, degree of steatosis, or cold ischemia time.[108] In an effort to address this issue, researchers from the University of Birmingham, United Kingdom, have developed an approach to assess the potential outcome of the recipient-donor pair, using artificial neural networks.[109] If these models prove useful, it is possible that, in the future, the allocation system might improve our ability to match a donor with the recipient who would be expected to have the best outcome. For now, however, the limited amount of donors and an ever-growing waiting list, will limit the application of such a system.

LIVING DONOR LIVER TRANSPLANTATION

Over the last decade, living donor liver transplantation (LDLT) using the right hepatic lobe of a healthy adult has become part of the armamentarium in a multitude of transplant centers around the world. This technique was initially developed in response to a worldwide organ shortage that resulted in increased waiting time and mortality on the transplant list.[52] In the United States, waiting list mortality was up to 25% in the late 1990s (UNOS/OPTN, www.optn.org, accessed November 2008), when the first 2 cases of adult-to-adult LDLT were performed at the University of Colorado in 1997.[110] Up to then, LDLT had been mainly reserved for adult-to-child transplantation, for which a smaller donor graft is needed, such that a less morbid operation, namely a left hepatectomy, can be performed.[111]

After the initial success, the number of LDLT procedures in the United States increased from 60 in 1996 (only 3 in adults), to 522 (411 adults) in 2001.[112] Several factors, including the much publicized death of a donor in New York, have resulted in a decline since then. At present, approximately 250 adult LDLT are performed annually in the United States, accounting for less than 4% of adult liver transplants (UNOS/OPTN, www.optn.org, accessed November 2008).

Advantages and Disadvantages of LDLT

The main advantage of LDLT is the ability to reduce the risk of dying while on the waiting list, especially for candidates who are not expected to obtain an organ in a timely fashion. Although the general indications are similar to deceased-donor liver transplantation (DDLT), recipients tend to have less advanced forms of liver disease as assessed by lower MELD scores at time of transplant, and generally suffer from HCC or complications of cirrhosis that are not necessarily taken into account when calculating the MELD score. Because LDLT is an elective procedure, it allows the transplant team to optimize the candidate's medical condition and to secure a "high quality" graft from a healthy individual.[52,113]

The main drawback to LDLT is the potential for harming an otherwise healthy individual, whose main motivation is the opportunity to save another person's life. Although most donors undergo uncomplicated hepatectomies, up to one third of patients suffer from postoperative complications and at least 3 donor deaths have been reported in the United States, with an estimated mortality of 0.2% to 0.4%.[114,115] Even so, most donors return to work after a mean of 10 weeks after surgery and no decline in health-related quality of life has been reported.[116–119] Most donors have an increased sense of self-esteem and family ties are often strengthened by the donation.[111]

Recipient and Donor Evaluation for LDLT

Most transplant centers performing LDLT in the United States will consider candidates who would also meet the standard UNOS DDLT listing criteria and as such undergo a similar pretransplant evaluation.

The donor candidates should be physically and mentally healthy adults who voluntarily express their desire to become liver donors. Once a potential donor has been identified, a thorough and stepwise evaluation is performed by a multidisciplinary team to ensure that the individual is a suitable candidate, that he/she is well informed about the risks and benefits of the procedure, and is making an autonomous and non-coerced decision.[113] Most donor candidates undergo a similar evaluation to the recipients, including noninvasive imaging studies of the liver to assess anatomic variants and adequacy of potential graft size, as this is a key factor in LDLT outcome. Another relevant variable in graft outcome is the degree of steatosis. To better assess liver steatosis in the potential donor, some transplant centers perform a biopsy in all the candidates, whereas others have more selective policies and only perform biopsies on those individuals who have increased BMI or signs of liver steatosis on imaging studies.[111,113] After this extensive evaluation, only 15% to 45% of subjects are considered suitable donor candidates and actually proceed to LDLT.[120,121]

LDLT Recipient Outcomes

After initial concerns about the efficacy of LDLT in adults, it has recently been demonstrated that in experienced centers, LDLT offers comparable outcomes to DDLT, even in recipients with HCC or hepatitis C.[122–128] In the United States, overall 1-, 3-, and 5-year patient survival rates for transplants performed from 1997 to 2004 was 86%, 78%, and 72% for DDLT, and 90%, 83%, and 78%, respectively, for LDLT (OPTN/UNOS, www.optn.org, accessed November 2008).

Other than the typical complications of a major surgical procedure, the main postoperative complications in LDLT recipients are biliary (15%–60%) and vascular in nature: bile leaks, biliary strictures, and right hepatic artery thrombosis.[129–132]

The transplanted right lobe and the remainder of the liver in the donor will regenerate rapidly, with more than 85% of the original hepatic volume restored within 1 week of surgery.[133] The regeneration and remodeling processes have been shown to continue for up to 1 year after LDLT[134,135] and are influenced by several factors, including severity of liver disease before transplantation and surgical technique.[113,136]

SUMMARY

Improved outcomes and increased availability have made liver transplantation the definitive therapeutic option for patients with end-stage liver disease. As most patients with liver disease are cared for by primary care providers, it is important for clinicians to be aware of the main indications and contraindications to transplantation, have a general understanding of the pretransplant evaluation process, and be able to refer patients to a transplant center in a timely fashion.

In recent years the organ allocation system in the United States has undergone modifications that have benefited patients awaiting liver transplantation. Further research in this area will certainly result in improvements in the current system. Living donor liver transplantation is now carried out in many transplant centers as a way to decrease mortality on the waiting list for selected candidates. This procedure poses unique clinical, technical, and ethical problems that will have to be resolved by the medical community.

REFERENCES

1. Ahmed A, Keeffe EB. Current indications and contraindications for liver transplantation. Clin Liver Dis 2007;11(2):227–47.
2. Tome S, Wells JT, Said A, et al. Quality of life after liver transplantation. A systematic review. J Hepatol 2008;48(4):567–77.
3. Kim WR, Brown RS Jr, Terrault NA, et al. Burden of liver disease in the United States: summary of a workshop. Hepatology 2002;36(1):227–42.
4. Olivera-Martinez MA, Gallegos-Orozco JF. Recurrent viral liver disease (hepatitis B and C) after liver transplantation. Arch Med Res 2007;38(6):691–701.
5. Sharma P, Lok A. Viral hepatitis and liver transplantation. Semin Liver Dis 2006; 26(3):285–97.
6. Roche B, Samuel D. Aspects of hepatitis C virus infection relating to liver transplantation. Eur J Gastroenterol Hepatol 2006;18(4):313–20.
7. Rodriguez-Luna H, Vargas HE. Management of hepatitis C virus infection in the setting of liver transplantation. Liver Transpl 2005;11(5):479–89.

8. Seeff LB, Miller RN, Rabkin CS, et al. 45-Year follow-up of hepatitis C virus infection in healthy young adults. Ann Intern Med 2000;132(2):105–11.

9. Befeler AS, Di Bisceglie AM. Hepatocellular carcinoma: diagnosis and treatment. Gastroenterology 2002;122(6):1609–19.

10. Murray KF, Carithers RL Jr. AASLD practice guidelines: evaluation of the patient for liver transplantation. Hepatology 2005;41(6):1407–32.

11. Berenguer M. Natural history of recurrent hepatitis C. Liver Transpl 2002;8(10 Suppl 1):S14–8.

12. Berenguer M, Ferrell L, Watson J, et al. HCV-related fibrosis progression following liver transplantation: increase in recent years. J Hepatol 2000;32(4):673–84.

13. Charlton M. Patient and graft survival following liver transplantation for hepatitis C: much ado about something. Gastroenterology 2002;122(4):1162–5.

14. Forman LM, Lewis JD, Berlin JA, et al. The association between hepatitis C infection and survival after orthotopic liver transplantation. Gastroenterology 2002;122(4):889–96.

15. Everson GT, Trotter J, Forman L, et al. Treatment of advanced hepatitis C with a low accelerating dosage regimen of antiviral therapy. Hepatology 2005; 42(2):255–62.

16. Verna EC, Brown RS Jr. Hepatitis C and liver transplantation: enhancing outcomes and should patients be retransplanted. Clin Liver Dis 2008;12(3): 637–59, ix–x.

17. Riediger C, Berberat PO, Sauer P, et al. Prophylaxis and treatment of recurrent viral hepatitis after liver transplantation. Nephrol Dial Transplant 2007;22(Suppl 8):viii37–46.

18. Triantos C, Samonakis D, Stigliano R, et al. Liver transplantation and hepatitis C virus: systematic review of antiviral therapy. Transplantation 2005;79(3):261–8.

19. Encke J, Kraus T, Mehrabi A, et al. Treatment of hepatitis C virus reinfection after liver transplantation. Transplantation 2005;80(1 Suppl):S125–7.

20. Borowsky SA, Strome S, Lott E. Continued heavy drinking and survival in alcoholic cirrhotics. Gastroenterology 1981;80(6):1405–9.

21. Powell WJ Jr, Klatskin G. Duration of survival in patients with Laennec's cirrhosis. Influence of alcohol withdrawal, and possible effects of recent changes in general management of the disease. Am J Med 1968;44(3):406–20.

22. Everhart JE, Beresford TP. Liver transplantation for alcoholic liver disease: a survey of transplantation programs in the United States. Liver Transpl Surg 1997;3(3):220–6.

23. Campbell DA Jr, Magee JC, Punch JD, et al. One center's experience with liver transplantation: alcohol use relapse over the long-term. Liver Transpl Surg 1998; 4(5 Suppl 1):S58–64.

24. Lucey MR. Is liver transplantation an appropriate treatment for acute alcoholic hepatitis? J Hepatol 2002;36(6):829–31.

25. Lucey MR. Liver transplantation for alcoholic liver disease. Clin Liver Dis 2007; 11(2):283–9.

26. Belle SH, Beringer KC, Detre KM. Liver transplantation for alcoholic liver disease in the United States: 1988 to 1995. Liver Transpl Surg 1997;3(3):212–9.

27. Pereira SP, Williams R. Liver transplantation for alcoholic liver disease at King's College Hospital: survival and quality of life. Liver Transpl Surg 1997;3(3): 245–50.

28. Roberts MS, Angus DC, Bryce CL, et al. Survival after liver transplantation in the United States: a disease-specific analysis of the UNOS database. Liver Transpl 2004;10(7):886–97.

29. Wiesner RH, Lombardero M, Lake JR, et al. Liver transplantation for end-stage alcoholic liver disease: an assessment of outcomes. Liver Transpl Surg 1997; 3(3):231–9.
30. Bellamy CO, DiMartini AM, Ruppert K, et al. Liver transplantation for alcoholic cirrhosis: long term follow-up and impact of disease recurrence. Transplantation 2001;72(4):619–26.
31. Lee RG. Recurrence of alcoholic liver disease after liver transplantation. Liver Transpl Surg 1997;3(3):292–5.
32. 2007 Annual report of the U.S. Organ Procurement and Transplantation Network and the Scientific Registry of Transplant Recipients: Transplant Data 1997-2006. Rockville (MD): Health Resources and Services Administration, Healthcare Systems Bureau, Division of Transplantation; 2007.
33. Heathcote EJ. Management of primary biliary cirrhosis. The American Association for the Study of Liver Diseases practice guidelines. Hepatology 2000;31(4): 1005–13.
34. Neuberger J. Liver transplantation for primary biliary cirrhosis: indications and risk of recurrence. J Hepatol 2003;39(2):142–8.
35. Liermann Garcia RF, Evangelista Garcia C, McMaster P, et al. Transplantation for primary biliary cirrhosis: retrospective analysis of 400 patients in a single center. Hepatology 2001;33(1):22–7.
36. Abu-Elmagd KM, Balan V, Abu-Elmagd KM, et al. Recurrent primary sclerosing cholangitis: from an academic illusion to a clinical reality [comment]. Liver Transpl 2005;11(11):1326–8.
37. Graziadei IW, Wiesner RH, Marotta PJ, et al. Long-term results of patients undergoing liver transplantation for primary sclerosing cholangitis. Hepatology 1999; 30(5):1121–7.
38. Goss JA, Shackleton CR, Farmer DG, et al. Orthotopic liver transplantation for primary sclerosing cholangitis. A 12-year single center experience. Ann Surg 1997;225(5):472–81 [discussion: 481–3].
39. Narumi S, Roberts JP, Emond JC, et al. Liver transplantation for sclerosing cholangitis. Hepatology 1995;22(2):451–7.
40. Maheshwari A, Yoo HY, Thuluvath PJ, et al. Long-term outcome of liver transplantation in patients with PSC: a comparative analysis with PBC. Am J Gastroenterol 2004;99(3):538–42.
41. Graziadei IW, Graziadei IW. Recurrence of primary sclerosing cholangitis after liver transplantation. Liver Transpl 2002;8(7):575–81.
42. Fabia R, Levy MF, Testa G, et al. Colon carcinoma in patients undergoing liver transplantation. Am J Surg 1998;176(3):265–9.
43. Loftus EV Jr, Aguilar HI, Sandborn WJ, et al. Risk of colorectal neoplasia in patients with primary sclerosing cholangitis and ulcerative colitis following orthotopic liver transplantation. Hepatology 1998;27(3):685–90.
44. El-Serag HB, Davila JA, Petersen NJ, et al. The continuing increase in the incidence of hepatocellular carcinoma in the United States: an update. Ann Intern Med 2003;139(10):817–23.
45. Hassan MM, Frome A, Patt YZ, et al. Rising prevalence of hepatitis C virus infection among patients recently diagnosed with hepatocellular carcinoma in the United States. J Clin Gastroenterol 2002;35(3):266–9.
46. El-Serag HB, Mason AC. Risk factors for the rising rates of primary liver cancer in the United States. Arch Intern Med 2000;160(21):3227–30.
47. Llovet JM, Schwartz M, Mazzaferro V. Resection and liver transplantation for hepatocellular carcinoma. Semin Liver Dis 2005;25(2):181–200.

48. Mazzaferro V, Chun YS, Poon RT, et al. Liver transplantation for hepatocellular carcinoma. Ann Surg Oncol 2008;15(4):1001–7.
49. Mazzaferro V, Regalia E, Doci R, et al. Liver transplantation for the treatment of small hepatocellular carcinomas in patients with cirrhosis. N Engl J Med 1996; 334(11):693–9.
50. Yoo HY, Patt CH, Geschwind JF, et al. The outcome of liver transplantation in patients with hepatocellular carcinoma in the United States between 1988 and 2001: 5-year survival has improved significantly with time. J Clin Oncol 2003; 21(23):4329–35.
51. Mazzaferro V. Results of liver transplantation: with or without Milan criteria? Liver Transpl 2007;13(11 Suppl 2):S44–7.
52. Everson GT, Membreno FE. Liver transplantation: indications, contraindications and results. In: Rodés J, Benhamou JP, Blei A, et al, editors. Textbook of hepatology: from basic science to clinical practice. 3rd edition. Oxford: Blackwell Publishing; 2007. p. 1984–95.
53. Sharma P, Rakela J. Management of pre-liver transplantation patients – part 1. Liver Transpl 2005;11(2):124–33.
54. Keswani RN, Ahmed A, Keeffe EB. Older age and liver transplantation: a review. Liver Transpl 2004;10(8):957–67.
55. Carey WD, Dumot JA, Pimentel RR, et al. The prevalence of coronary artery disease in liver transplant candidates over age 50. Transplantation 1995;59(6):859–64.
56. Donovan CL, Marcovitz PA, Punch JD, et al. Two-dimensional and dobutamine stress echocardiography in the preoperative assessment of patients with end-stage liver disease prior to orthotopic liver transplantation. Transplantation 1996;61(8):1180–8.
57. Keeffe EB. Summary of guidelines on organ allocation and patient listing for liver transplantation. Liver Transpl Surg 1998;4(5 Suppl 1):S108–14.
58. Keeffe EB. Update on liver transplantation. Rev Gastroenterol Mex 2004; 69(Suppl 3):160–70.
59. Krowka MJ. Hepatopulmonary syndrome: recent literature (1997 to 1999) and implications for liver transplantation. Liver Transpl 2000;6(4 Suppl 1):S31–5.
60. Krowka MJ. Hepatopulmonary syndrome and portopulmonary hypertension: implications for liver transplantation. Clin Chest Med 2005;26(4):587–97, vi.
61. Arguedas MR, Abrams GA, Krowka MJ, et al. Prospective evaluation of outcomes and predictors of mortality in patients with hepatopulmonary syndrome undergoing liver transplantation. Hepatology 2003;37(1):192–7.
62. Krowka MJ, Porayko MK, Plevak DJ, et al. Hepatopulmonary syndrome with progressive hypoxemia as an indication for liver transplantation: case reports and literature review. Mayo Clin Proc 1997;72(1):44–53.
63. Colle IO, Moreau R, Godinho E, et al. Diagnosis of portopulmonary hypertension in candidates for liver transplantation: a prospective study. Hepatology 2003; 37(2):401–9.
64. Mucke HA. Pulmonary arterial hypertension: on the way to a manageable disease. Curr Opin Investig Drugs 2008;9(9):957–62.
65. Ramsay MA. Portopulmonary hypertension and hepatopulmonary syndrome, and liver transplantation. Int Anesthesiol Clin 2006;44(3):69–82.
66. Nair S, Verma S, Thuluvath PJ. Pretransplant renal function predicts survival in patients undergoing orthotopic liver transplantation. Hepatology 2002;35(5): 1179–85.
67. Lafayette RA, Pare G, Schmid CH, et al. Pretransplant renal dysfunction predicts poorer outcome in liver transplantation. Clin Nephrol 1997;48(3):159–64.

68. Storm C, Bernhardt WM, Schaeffner E, et al. Immediate recovery of renal function after orthotopic liver transplantation in a patient with hepatorenal syndrome requiring hemodialysis for more than 8 months. Transplant Proc 2007;39(2):544–6.
69. Richardson D, Stoves J, Davies MH, et al. Liver transplantation for dialysis dependent hepatorenal failure. Nephrol Dial Transplant 1999;14(11):2742–5.
70. Martin-Llahi M, Pepin MN, Guevara M, et al. Terlipressin and albumin vs albumin in patients with cirrhosis and hepatorenal syndrome: a randomized study. Gastroenterology 2008;134(5):1352–9.
71. Sanyal AJ, Boyer T, Garcia-Tsao G, et al. A randomized, prospective, double-blind, placebo-controlled trial of terlipressin for type 1 hepatorenal syndrome. Gastroenterology 2008;134(5):1360–8.
72. Nair S, Verma S, Thuluvath PJ. Obesity and its effect on survival in patients undergoing orthotopic liver transplantation in the United States. Hepatology 2002;35(1):105–9.
73. John PR, Thuluvath PJ. Outcome of liver transplantation in patients with diabetes mellitus: a case-control study. Hepatology 2001;34(5):889–95.
74. Shields PL, Tang H, Neuberger JM, et al. Poor outcome in patients with diabetes mellitus undergoing liver transplantation. Transplantation 1999;68(4):530–5.
75. Neff GW, Sherman KE, Eghtesad B, et al. Review article: current status of liver transplantation in HIV-infected patients. Aliment Pharmacol Ther 2004;20(10): 993–1000.
76. Roland ME, Adey D, Carlson LL, et al. Kidney and liver transplantation in HIV-infected patients: case presentations and review. AIDS Patient Care STDS 2003; 17(10):501–7.
77. Roland ME, Stock PG. Liver transplantation in HIV-infected recipients. Semin Liver Dis 2006;26(3):273–84.
78. Ahmed A, Keeffe EB. Pretransplant evaluation and care. In: Boyer TD, Wright TL, Manns MP, editors. Zakim and Boyer's hepatology: a textbook of liver disease. 5th edition. Philadelphia: Saunders Elsevier; 2006. p. 933–45.
79. Manzanet G, Sanjuan F, Orbis P, et al. Liver transplantation in patients with portal vein thrombosis. Liver Transpl 2001;7(2):125–31.
80. Yerdel MA, Gunson B, Mirza D, et al. Portal vein thrombosis in adults undergoing liver transplantation: risk factors, screening, management, and outcome. Transplantation 2000;69(9):1873–81.
81. Fattovich G, Giustina G, Degos F, et al. Morbidity and mortality in compensated cirrhosis type C: a retrospective follow-up study of 384 patients. Gastroenterology 1997;112(2):463–72.
82. Freeman RBJ. Selection and timing of liver transplantation. In: Schiff ER, Sorrel MF, Maddrey WC, editors. Schiff's diseases of the liver. 10th edition. Philadelphia: Lippincott Williams & Wilkins; 2007. p. 1453–65.
83. Consensus conference: Indications for Liver Transplantation, January 19 and 20, 2005, Lyon-Palais Des Congres: text of recommendations (long version). Liver Transpl 2006;12(6):998–1011.
84. [Consensus document of the Spanish Society of Liver Transplantation]. Gastroenterol Hepatol 2008;31(2):82–91 [in Spanish].
85. Koffron A, Stein JA. Liver transplantation: indications, pretransplant evaluation, surgery, and posttransplant complications. Med Clin North Am 2008;92(4): 861–88, ix.
86. Plotkin JS, Benitez RM, Kuo PC, et al. Dobutamine stress echocardiography for preoperative cardiac risk stratification in patients undergoing orthotopic liver transplantation. Liver Transpl Surg 1998;4(4):253–7.

87. Plotkin JS, Johnson LB, Rustgi V, et al. Coronary artery disease and liver transplantation: the state of the art. Liver Transpl 2000;6(4 Suppl 1):S53–6.

88. Freeman RB Jr. The model for end-stage liver disease comes of age. Clin Liver Dis 2007;11(2):249–63.

89. Wiesner RH. Patient selection in an era of donor liver shortage: current US policy. Nat Clin Pract Gastroenterol Hepatol 2005;2(1):24–30.

90. Gish RG. Do we need to MEND the MELD? Liver Transpl 2007;13(4):486–7.

91. Pugh RN, Murray-Lyon IM, Dawson JL, et al. Transection of the oesophagus for bleeding oesophageal varices. Br J Surg 1973;60(8):646–9.

92. Malinchoc M, Kamath PS, Gordon FD, et al. A model to predict poor survival in patients undergoing transjugular intrahepatic portosystemic shunts. Hepatology 2000;31(4):864–71.

93. Kamath PS, Wiesner RH, Malinchoc M, et al. A model to predict survival in patients with end-stage liver disease. Hepatology 2001;33(2):464–70.

94. Salerno F, Merli M, Cazzaniga M, et al. MELD score is better than Child-Pugh score in predicting 3-month survival of patients undergoing transjugular intrahepatic portosystemic shunt. J Hepatol 2002;36(4):494–500.

95. Wiesner R, Edwards E, Freeman R, et al. Model for end-stage liver disease (MELD) and allocation of donor livers. Gastroenterology 2003;124(1):91–6.

96. McDiarmid SV, Anand R, Lindblad AS. Development of a pediatric end-stage liver disease score to predict poor outcome in children awaiting liver transplantation. Transplantation 2002;74(2):173–81.

97. Freeman RB Jr, Wiesner RH, Harper A, et al. The new liver allocation system: moving toward evidence-based transplantation policy. Liver Transpl 2002;8(9):851–8.

98. Freeman RB, Wiesner RH, Edwards E, et al. Results of the first year of the new liver allocation plan. Liver Transpl 2004;10(1):7–15.

99. Merion RM, Rush SH, Dykstra DM, et al. Predicted lifetimes for adult and pediatric split liver versus adult whole liver transplant recipients. Am J Transplant 2004;4(11):1792–7.

100. Wiesner RH. Evidence-based evolution of the MELD/PELD liver allocation policy. Liver Transpl 2005;11(3):261–3.

101. Freeman RB, Gish RG, Harper A, et al. Model for end-stage liver disease (MELD) exception guidelines: results and recommendations from the MELD exception study group and conference (MESSAGE) for the approval of patients who need liver transplantation with diseases not considered by the standard MELD formula. Liver Transpl 2006;12(12 Suppl 3):S128–36.

102. Cholongitas E, Marelli L, Shusang V, et al. A systematic review of the performance of the model for end-stage liver disease (MELD) in the setting of liver transplantation. Liver Transpl 2006;12(7):1049–61.

103. Cholongitas E, Papatheodoridis GV, Vangeli M, et al. Systematic review: the model for end-stage liver disease—should it replace Child-Pugh's classification for assessing prognosis in cirrhosis? Aliment Pharmacol Ther 2005;22(11–12):1079–89.

104. Biggins SW, Rodriguez HJ, Bacchetti P, et al. Serum sodium predicts mortality in patients listed for liver transplantation. Hepatology 2005;41(1):32–9.

105. Heuman DM, Abou-Assi SG, Habib A, et al. Persistent ascites and low serum sodium identify patients with cirrhosis and low MELD scores who are at high risk for early death. Hepatology 2004;40(4):802–10.

106. Ruf AE, Kremers WK, Chavez LL, et al. Addition of serum sodium into the MELD score predicts waiting list mortality better than MELD alone. Liver Transpl 2005;11(3):336–43.

107. Stewart CA, Malinchoc M, Kim WR, et al. Hepatic encephalopathy as a predictor of survival in patients with end-stage liver disease. Liver Transpl 2007;13(10):1366–71.
108. Lucey MR. How will patients be selected for transplantation in the future? Liver Transpl 2004;10(10 Suppl 2):S90–2.
109. Haydon GH, Hiltunen Y, Lucey MR, et al. Self-organizing maps can determine outcome and match recipients and donors at orthotopic liver transplantation. Transplantation 2005;79(2):213–8.
110. Wachs ME, Bak TE, Karrer FM, et al. Adult living donor liver transplantation using a right hepatic lobe. Transplantation 1998;66(10):1313–6.
111. Florman S, Miller CM. Live donor liver transplantation. Liver Transpl 2006;12(4): 499–510.
112. Brown RS Jr, Russo MW, Lai M, et al. A survey of liver transplantation from living adult donors in the United States. N Engl J Med 2003;348(9):818–25.
113. Brown RS Jr. Live donors in liver transplantation. Gastroenterology 2008;134(6): 1802–13.
114. Renz JF, Busuttil RW. Adult-to-adult living-donor liver transplantation: a critical analysis. Semin Liver Dis 2000;20(4):411–24.
115. Tuttle-Newhall JE, Collins BH, Desai DM, et al. The current status of living donor liver transplantation. Curr Probl Surg 2005;42(3):144–83.
116. Kim-Schluger L, Florman SS, Schiano T, et al. Quality of life after lobectomy for adult liver transplantation. Transplantation 2002;73(10):1593–7.
117. Miyagi S, Kawagishi N, Fujimori K, et al. Risks of donation and quality of donors' life after living donor liver transplantation. Transpl Int 2005;18(1):47–51.
118. Trotter JF, Talamantes M, McClure M, et al. Right hepatic lobe donation for living donor liver transplantation: impact on donor quality of life. Liver Transpl 2001; 7(6):485–93.
119. Chan SC, Liu CL, Lo CM, et al. Donor quality of life before and after adult-to-adult right liver live donor liver transplantation. Liver Transpl 2006;12(10):1529–36.
120. Trotter JF, Campsen J, Bak T, et al. Outcomes of donor evaluations for adult-to-adult right hepatic lobe living donor liver transplantation. Am J Transplant 2006; 6(8):1882–9.
121. Trotter JF, Wisniewski KA, Terrault NA, et al. Outcomes of donor evaluation in adult-to-adult living donor liver transplantation. Hepatology 2007;46(5):1476–84.
122. Berg CL, Gillespie BW, Merion RM, et al. Improvement in survival associated with adult-to-adult living donor liver transplantation. Gastroenterology 2007; 133(6):1806–13.
123. Fisher RA, Kulik LM, Freise CE, et al. Hepatocellular carcinoma recurrence and death following living and deceased donor liver transplantation. Am J Transplant 2007;7(6):1601–8.
124. Guo L, Orrego M, Rodriguez-Luna H, et al. Living donor liver transplantation for hepatitis C-related cirrhosis: no difference in histological recurrence when compared to deceased donor liver transplantation recipients. Liver Transpl 2006;12(4):560–5.
125. Kulik L, Abecassis M. Living donor liver transplantation for hepatocellular carcinoma. Gastroenterology 2004;127(5 Suppl 1):S277–82.
126. Lo CM, Fan ST, Liu CL, et al. Living donor versus deceased donor liver transplantation for early irresectable hepatocellular carcinoma. Br J Surg 2007; 94(1):78–86.
127. Shiffman ML, Stravitz RT, Contos MJ, et al. Histologic recurrence of chronic hepatitis C virus in patients after living donor and deceased donor liver transplantation. Liver Transpl 2004;10(10):1248–55.

128. Terrault NA, Berenguer M. Treating hepatitis C infection in liver transplant recipients. Liver Transpl 2006;12(8):1192–204.
129. Bak T, Wachs M, Trotter J, et al. Adult-to-adult living donor liver transplantation using right-lobe grafts: results and lessons learned from a single-center experience. Liver Transpl 2001;7(8):680–6.
130. Fan ST. Live donor liver transplantation in adults. Transplantation 2006;82(6): 723–32.
131. Ghobrial RM, Saab S, Lassman C, et al. Donor and recipient outcomes in right lobe adult living donor liver transplantation. Liver Transpl 2002;8(10):901–9.
132. Miller CM, Gondolesi GE, Florman S, et al. One hundred nine living donor liver transplants in adults and children: a single-center experience. Ann Surg 2001; 234(3):301–11 [discussion: 311–2].
133. Marcos A, Fisher RA, Ham JM, et al. Liver regeneration and function in donor and recipient after right lobe adult to adult living donor liver transplantation. Transplantation 2000;69(7):1375–9.
134. Kawasaki S, Makuuchi M, Ishizone S, et al. Liver regeneration in recipients and donors after transplantation. Lancet 1992;339(8793):580–1.
135. Nakagami M, Morimoto T, Itoh K, et al. Patterns of restoration of remnant liver volume after graft harvesting in donors for living related liver transplantation. Transplant Proc 1998;30(1):195–9.
136. Akamatsu N, Sugawara Y, Kaneko J, et al. Effects of middle hepatic vein reconstruction on right liver graft regeneration. Transplantation 2003;76(5):832–7.

Index

Note: Page numbers of article titles are in **boldface** type.

Med Clin N Am 93 (2009) 951–962
doi:10.1016/S0025-7125(09)00082-0
0025-7125/09/$ – see front matter © 2009 Elsevier Inc. All rights reserved.

medical.theclinics.com